CONTENTS

INTRODUCTION

Ninja Foodi Grill: overview

The Ninja Foodi 5-in-1 Indoor Grill is an incredible multi-purpose cooking machine. It can air fry, roast, bake, dehydrate and grill indoors. It won't do your laundry or wash your car, but it does seem to do everything else. Meats, vegetables, and even fruit come out with juicy perfection. You can also use the Ninja Foodi 5-in-1 Indoor Grill to make dried fruit and beef jerky snacks.

Ninja Foodi 5-In-1 Indoor Grill: Notable Features

This multifunctional kitchen appliance can air fry, roast, bake, dehydrate and grill indoors. The amount of smoke produced is minimal so you can use it inside a kitchen or small apartment. The Ninja Foodi comes in either back or silver, both of which look sleek and modern.

Pros

Cooks with minimal smoking

Air fry crisp

1760-watt— the same BTU as an outdoor cooking unit

Dishwasher safe components

Cons

The closed lid makes it hard to see how the food is cooking inside

Grilling Meats to Perfection

Even though it is multi-purposed, the raison d'être for this cooking machine is the grilling. The Ninja Foodi nicely sears steaks to perfection while draining away the fat. Users reported that their sirloin steaks came out perfectly seared, juicy and delectable. Hamburgers come out the best, but you will achieve the best results when steaming the meat before grilling.

With the air recirculation on, the Ninja Foodi works as an air fryer. French fries will come out soft and crispy, but with a lot less oil than a traditional deep fryer. It is an utterly convenient way to cook mahi mahi fish filets and salmon steaks. Cover yours with green onions and lemon juice to prevent them being over-dried.

With most components being dishwasher safe, cleanup will be a snap. Everything can be broken down and tossed in the lower dishwasher rack.

Roasting, Baking & Dehydrating

The Ninja Foodi excels as a vegetable roaster. Roasting zucchini, tomatoes and brussel sprouts will be effortless. The recirculating air essentially turns this grill into a convection oven.

The Ninja Foodi is excellent for dehydrating fruit. Don't know what to do with those bargain fruits you picked up at the farmer's market? Slice those extra summer fruits, toss them into the machine and save them for the winter.

Smoke Reduction

The Ninja Foodi is advertised as an indoor grill and they don't claim that it is entirely smokeless. Some people have noticed that when cooking some types of drier meats or butter some smoke did manage to escape the internal venting system. Don't get me wrong, the amount of smoke produced is significantly less than other countertop grills. Fundamental physics is at work here, and the hot gasses have to go somewhere. We don't think any design could do this job correctly. We recommend using the Ninja Foodi 5-in-1 Indoor Grill with some kind of ventilation.

Now that we have an overview of how the Ninja Foodi Grill we can dive into the sea of recipes, are you ready? Let's start!

BREAKFAST RECIPES

1. Almond Muffins

Servings: 6
Cooking Time: 25 Minutes
Ingredients:

- 8 Tbsp butter
- ½ cup Baking Stevia
- 1 egg
- 1 tsp vanilla
- 2 cups coconut flour
- 2 tsp baking powder
- 1 tsp salt
- ½ cup chopped almonds
- ½ cup buttermilk

Directions:

1. Use an electric mixer to cream the butter and stevia together until they are light and fluffy.
2. Mix the vanilla and eggs in a small bowl then add to the mixer with the butter blend. Mix until just combined
3. Add the remaining dry ingredients to the mixer and fold together by hand. Add the buttermilk and mix until smooth.
4. Add the almonds to the batter and mix briefly.
5. Pour the muffin batter into eight silicone muffin cups. Place the muffin cups inside the Ninja Foodi on top of a metal trivet.
6. Press the air crisp button and set the temperature to 350 degrees and program the timer to 25 minutes.
7. Once cooked, a toothpick should come out of the center of the cake cleanly. Allow to cool and serve.
- **Nutrition Info:** Calories: 2386g, Carbohydrates: 29g, Protein: 6g, Fat: 26g, Sugar: 5g, Sodium: 699 g

2. Cheesy Hash

Servings: 6
Cooking Time: 30 Minutes
Ingredients:

- 6 eggs
- 4 cups riced cauliflower
- ¼ cup milk
- 1 onion, chopped
- 3 Tbsp butter
- 1 ½ cups cheddar cheese

Directions:

1. Press the saute button on your Ninja Foodi and add the butter and the onions. Cook, stirring occasionally until the onions are soft, about 5 minutes.
2. Add the iced cauliflower to the pot and stir. Turn on the air crisper for 15 minutes, turning the cauliflower halfway through.
3. In a small bowl, mix the eggs and milk together then pour over the browned cauliflower.
4. Sprinkle the cheddar cheese on top and close the lid of the Ninja Foodi for one minute to just melt the cheese. Serve while hot
- **Nutrition Info:** Calories: 291g, Carbohydrates: 8g, Protein: 18g, Fat: 22 g, Sugar: 1g, Sodium: 729g

3. Coconut Oatmeal

Servings:6
Cooking Time: 10 Minutes
Ingredients:

- 1 cup shredded dried coconut flakes
- 3 cups coconut milk
- 3 cups water
- ¼ cup psyllium husks
- ½ cup coconut flour
- 1 ½ tsp vanilla extract
- ½ tsp cinnamon
- ½ cup granulated stevia

Directions:

1. Add all of the ingredients into the Ninja Foodi and stir together briefly
2. Place the lid on and set the steamer valve to seal. Set the pressure cooker function to 1 minute (it will take about 10 minutes to come to pressure).
3. When the oatmeal is done, do a quick pressure release by opening the steamer valve carefully. Serve while hot
- **Nutrition Info:** Calories: 202g, Carbohydrates: 6g , Protein: 3g, Fat: 16g, Sugar: 2g, Sodium: 52 g

4. Blackberry Muffins

Servings: 6
Cooking Time: 25 Minutes
Ingredients:
- 8 Tbsp butter
- ½ cup Baking Stevia
- 1 egg
- 1 tsp vanilla
- 2 cups coconut flour
- 2 tsp baking powder
- 1 tsp salt
- 1 cup fresh blackberries
- ½ cup buttermilk

Directions:
1. Use an electric mixer to cream the butter and stevia together until they are light and fluffy.
2. Mix the vanilla and eggs in a small bowl then add to the mixer with the butter blend. Mix until just combined
3. In a separate bowl, toss the blackberries and ¼ cup almond flour to coat the berries.
4. Add the remaining dry ingredients to the mixer and fold together by hand. Add the buttermilk and mix until smooth.
5. Add the blackberries to the batter and mix briefly.
6. Pour the muffin batter into eight silicone muffin cups. Place the muffin cups inside the Ninja Foodi on top of a metal trivet.
7. Press the air crisp button and set the temperature to 350 degrees and program the timer to 25 minutes.
8. Once cooked, a toothpick should come out of the center of the cake cleanly. Allow to cool and serve.
- **Nutrition Info:** Calories: 285g, Carbohydrates: 2g , Protein: 6g, Fat: 17g, Sugar: 3g, Sodium: 590 g

5. Sausage Solo

Servings: 4
Cooking Time: 35 Minutes
Ingredients:
- 4 eggs
- 4 cooked and sliced sausages
- 2 tbsps. butter
- ½ c. grated mozzarella cheese
- ½ c. cream

Directions:
1. Mix together eggs and cream in a bowl and beat well.
2. Put the egg mixture in the pot of Ninja Foodi and top evenly with cheese and sausage slices.
3. Press "Bake/Roast" and set the timer to 20 minutes at 345 degrees F.
4. Dish out after 20 minutes and serve immediately.
- **Nutrition Info:** 180 calories, 12.7g fat, 3.9g carbs, 12.4g protein

6. Breakfast Stuffed Baked Potatoes

Servings: 4 Servings
Cooking Time: 8 Hours 10 Minutes
Ingredients:
- 4 potatoes, scrubbed and pricked all over
- 4 strips bacon, cooked and crumbled
- 4 eggs
- ½ cup cheddar cheese, grated
- 1 avocado, sliced
- ¼ cup chives, chopped
- 1 teaspoon olive oil
- Salt & pepper

Directions:
1. Rub the potatoes with oil and sprinkle with salt and pepper. Wrap in foil and place them in the cooking pot. Lock the lid in place and select slow cooking function on low heat. Cook potatoes overnight.
2. In the morning, carefully remove the potatoes and set the cooker to saute on med-high heat. Cook bacon till crisp, drain on paper towel and crumble when cool enough to do so.
3. Fry the eggs how you like them.
4. To assemble, cut the potatoes open, sprinkle cheese over them. Top with bacon, an egg, a slice of avocado and the chives. Salt and pepper to taste and enjoy.

7. Bacon And Egg Hash

Servings: 6
Cooking Time: 30 Minutes
Ingredients:

- 6 eggs
- 4 cups riced cauliflower
- ¼ cup milk
- 1 cup crumbled, cooked bacon
- 1 onion, chopped
- 3 Tbsp butter
- ½ cups cheddar cheese

Directions:

1. Press the saute button on your Ninja Foodi and add the butter and the onions. Cook, stirring occasionally until the onions are soft, about 5 minutes.
2. Add the riced cauliflower to the pot and stir. Turn on the air crisper for 15 minutes, turning the cauliflower halfway through.
3. In a small bowl, mix the eggs and milk together then pour over the browned cauliflower.
4. Sprinkle the cheddar cheese on top and close the lid of the Ninja Foodi for one minute to just melt the cheese. Serve while hot
- **Nutrition Info:** Calories: 301g, Carbohydrates: 3g, Protein: 18g, Fat: 26 g, Sugar: 1g, Sodium: 595g

8. Double Meat Breakfast Casserole

Servings: 4 -6 Servings
Cooking Time: 50 Minutes
Ingredients:

- ½ pound breakfast sausage
- 2 cups hash browns, shredded and thawed
- 4 slices bacon, chopped
- 6 eggs
- ¾ cup Velveeta, cubed
- ½ cup cheddar cheese, grated
- ½ cup mushrooms, sliced
- ¼ cup red bell pepper, chopped
- ¼ cup green bell pepper, chopped
- ¼ cup onion, chopped fine
- 2 -3 tablespoons sour cream

Directions:

1. Set the cooker to saute on med-high heat. Add the sausage and cook till brown. Remove with a slotted spoon and set aside.
2. Add bacon and cook, the remove it and set aside too. Drain all but 2 tablespoons of fat from the cooking pot.

3. Add vegetables and hash browns to the pot and cook till vegetables soften, stirring often. Stir in Velveeta cheese and continue cooking till it is melted and combined.
4. Meanwhile, in a large mixing bowl, whisk together eggs, sour cream, cheddar cheese and cooked bacon together.
5. Once the Velveeta is melted, top with sausage then pour the egg mixture over that.
6. Lock the Tender Crisp lid in place and set the temperature to 350 degrees. Bake the casserole for 35 -40 minutes or the center is set. Let rest 10 minutes before serving.

9. Cheesy Ham & Egg Casserole

Servings: 8 Servings
Cooking Time: 4 -8 Hours
Ingredients:

- 1 bag O'Brien potatoes, frozen
- 1 dozen eggs
- ½ pound ham, diced
- 1 cup cheddar cheese, grated
- ½ cup milk
- Salt & pepper

Directions:

1. Lightly spray the inside of the cooking pot with cooking spray.
2. Place the potatoes in the pot. Then top with ham and the cheese.
3. Beat the eggs in a large bowl. Stir in milk, salt and pepper and pour over the other ingredients.
4. Secure the lid and select slow cooker function. The casserole will be done in 4 hours on high heat or 8 hours on low.

10. Almond Spice Oatmeal

Servings: 6
Cooking Time: 10 Minutes
Ingredients:

- 1 ½ cups chopped almonds
- 3 cups almond milk
- 2 cups water
- ½ cup psyllium husks
- 1 ½ tsp vanilla extract
- ½ tsp cinnamon
- ¼ tsp nutmeg
- ½ cup granulated stevia

Directions:

1. Add all of the ingredients into the Ninja Foodi and stir together briefly
2. Place the lid on and set the steamer valve to seal. Set the pressure cooker function to 1 minute (it will take about 10 minutes to come to pressure).
3. When the oatmeal is done, do a quick pressure release by opening the steamer valve carefully. Serve while hot
- **Nutrition Info:** Calories: 136g, Carbohydrates: 3g, Protein: 4g, Fat: 9g, Sugar: 1g, Sodium: 66 g

11. Strawberries & Cream Quinoa

Servings: 3-4 Servings
Cooking Time: 8 Hours
Ingredients:
- 2 cups milk
- 1 ½ cups strawberries, halved
- 1 cup dry quinoa, rinsed
- 1 medium banana, sliced
- 2 tablespoons butter
- Honey to taste

Directions:

1. Add all ingredients to cooking pot and stir to combine.
2. Secure the lid and select slow cooking function on low heat. Cook 6 – 8 hours.
3. Serve warm topped with honey.

12. Easy Glazed Doughnuts

Servings: 8 Doughnuts & 8 Doughnut Holes
Cooking Time: 5 Mins
Ingredients:
- 2 cups flour
- ½ cup milk, room temperature
- ¼ cup sugar
- 1 egg, beaten
- 2 tablespoons butter, melted
- 1 ½ teaspoons fast acting yeast
- ¼ teaspoon nutmeg, optional
- salt
- Glaze:
- 1 cup powdered sugar
- 4 teaspoons water
- candy sprinkles

Directions:

1. Combine dry ingredients in a large bowl. Stir in milk, butter and egg to form a soft dough.
2. Transfer dough to a lightly floured surface and knead 2-3 minutes till smooth. Place the dough in a lightly oiled bowl, cover and let rise in a warm place till double in size, about 30 minutes.
3. Turn dough out onto a lightly floured surface and roll out to 1/4-inch thickness. Cut out 8 doughnuts using a 3-inch round cutter. Then use a 1-inch round cutter to remove center.
4. Leave the doughnuts and holes on the lightly floured surface and loosely cover with a cloth, let rise till double again.
5. Lightly spray the basket with cooking spray. Place half the doughnuts in the basket, in a single layer. Secure the Tender Crisp lid and set the temperature to 350 degrees. Cook 4 -5 minutes till golden brown. Repeat
6. To make the glaze, whisk the powdered sugar and water together till thoroughly mixed. Dip the doughnuts and holes in the glaze and place on a wire rack. Top with candy sprinkles. Let set about 10 minutes, till glaze hardens, then serve.

13. Cauliflower Hash Browns

Servings: 6
Cooking Time: 30 Minutes
Ingredients:
- 6 eggs
- 4 cups riced cauliflower
- ¼ cup milk
- 1 onion, chopped
- 3 Tbsp butter
- 1 ½ cups chopped, cooked ham
- ½ cup shredded cheese

Directions:

1. Press the saute button on your Ninja Foodi and add the butter and the onions. Cook, stirring occasionally until the onions are soft, about 5 minutes.
2. Add the iced cauliflower to the pot and stir. Turn on the air crisper for 15 minutes, turning the cauliflower halfway through.

3. In a small bowl, mix the eggs and milk together then pour over the browned cauliflower.
4. Sprinkle the ham over the top of the egg mix.
5. Press the air crisp button again and set the timer for 10 minutes.
6. Sprinkle the cheddar cheese on top and close the lid of the Ninja Foodi for one minute to just melt the cheese. Serve while hot
- **Nutrition Info:** Calories: 166g, Carbohydrates: 3g, Protein: 9g, Fat: 14 g, Sugar: 1g, Sodium: 278 g

14. Cherry Fritters

Servings: 12 Fritters
Cooking Time: 30 Minutes
Ingredients:
- 2 ¾ cups flour
- 1 ¼ cups sweet cherries, pitted and chopped
- 1 cup milk
- 1 egg
- 3 tablespoons sugar
- 2 tablespoons butter, soft
- 2 ¼ teaspoons instant yeast
- 1 teaspoon vanilla
- ½ teaspoon salt
- ½ teaspoon almond extract
- Glaze
- 1 ¼ cups powdered sugar
- 3 tablespoons milk
- 1 teaspoon vanilla extract
- ½ teaspoon almond extract

Directions:
1. Make the dough the night before. In a large bowl, mix flour, sugar, yeast and salt together. Beat in milk, butter, extracts and egg till dough forms.
2. Transfer dough to a lightly floured surface and knead about 6 minutes. Place the dough into a buttered bowl and cover with plastic. Chill overnight.
3. Next day, transfer dough to a well-floured work surface. Press into a rectangle about 12 x 8 inches. Sprinkle the cherries over the dough being sure to leave about ½ inch at the edges plain. Roll up along the widest

side. Slice into 12 pieces, place on flour dusted, line cookie sheet and loosely cover. Let rise for 20-30 minutes or till double in size.
4. Lightly spray the rolls with cooking spray, then add 2 at a time to the fryer basket. Place in the cooker and secure the Tender Crisp lid. Set the temperature for 360 degrees and cook 1 -2 minutes on each side, or till they are golden brown. Remove to a wire rack and repeat with remaining rolls.
5. Whisk the glaze ingredients together in a medium bowl. Dip the top of each fritter in glaze then place back on the rack. Allow several minutes for the glaze to set before serving.

15. Onion Tofu Scramble

Servings: 4
Cooking Time: 8 Minutes
Ingredients:
- 4 tbsps. butter
- 2 blocks tofu, cubed
- Salt and black pepper
- 1 c. grated cheddar cheese
- 2 medium sliced onions

Directions:
1. Mix together tofu, salt and black pepper in a bowl.
2. Press "Sauté" on Ninja Foodi and add butter and onions.
3. Sauté for about 3 minutes and add seasoned tofu.
4. Cook for about 2 minutes and add cheddar cheese.
5. Lock the lid and set the Ninja Foodi on "Air Crisp" for about 3 minutes at 340 degrees F.
6. Dish out in a serving plate and serve hot.
- **Nutrition Info:** 184 calories, 12.7g fat, 6.3g carbs, 12.2g protein

16. Bacon, Avocado And Cheese

Servings: 4
Cooking Time: 7 Minutes
Ingredients:
- 8 slices bacon
- 2 Avocados, sliced
- ½ cup cheddar cheese

- ¼ tsp ground black pepper

Directions:
1. Prepare a baking pan that fits in your Ninja Foodi bowl by greasing the pan with butter. Set aside
2. Lay the bacon strips inside the Ninja Foodi, trying not to layer them on top of each other.
3. Set the Ninja Foodi to air crisp at 325 for 7 minutes.
4. Remove the pan of bacon from the Ninja Foodi and place the sliced avocado on top. Sprinkle the top with the cheese and with the ground black pepper. Return to the Foodi and cook for another 2 minutes to melt the cheese. Remove and enjoy while hot!
- **Nutrition Info:** Calories: 265g, Carbohydrates: 8g , Protein: 10g, Fat: 23g, Sugar: 2g, Sodium: 431 g

17. Almond French Toast

Servings: 4
Cooking Time: 7 Minutes
Ingredients:
- 6 eggs
- 1 cup milk
- 4 cups keto almond bread, cut in cubes
- ¼ tsp salt
- 1 tsp vanilla extract
- ½ tsp cinnamon

Directions:
1. Prepare a baking pan that fits in your Ninja Foodi bowl by greasing the pan with butter. Set aside
2. In a medium bowl, whisk together the eggs, milk, salt, vanilla and cinnamon and then add the almond bread to the bowl and stir briefly. Let sit for one hour
3. Pour the egg mix into the prepared baking pan and lower the pan into the Ninja Foodi.
4. Set the Ninja Foodi to air crisp at 325 for 18 minutes.
5. Remove the pan of French toast from the Ninja Foodi and enjoy while hot!
- **Nutrition Info:** Calories: 220g, Carbohydrates: 8g , Protein: 22g, Fat: 11g, Sugar: 5g, Sodium:708 g

18. Bacon And Egg Bites

Servings: 6
Cooking Time: 20 Minutes
Ingredients:
- 5 slices bacon
- ½ cup milk
- 1 cup chopped spinach
- 6 eggs

Directions:
1. Place the bacon strips in the Ninja Foodi air crisper basket and use the air crisp function, set for 10 minutes to cook the bacon. Remove the basket and the strips and pour the bacon grease into a separate small bowl.
2. Add the eggs to the bacon grease along with the spinach, crumbled cooked bacon and milk.
3. Spray an egg bite mold and pour the egg mix evenly into each mold. Place the mold on top of the metal trivet inside the Ninja Foodi. Lower the crisper lid and set the temperature for 375 for 17 minutes.
4. Once cooked, remove the egg mold from the Ninja Foodi and let cool. Pop the egg bites out of the mold and serve hot or cold.
- **Nutrition Info:** Calories: 118g, Carbohydrates: 2g , Protein: 9g, Fat: 8 g, Sugar: 2g, Sodium: 216 g

19. Bacon Veggies Combo

Servings: 4
Cooking Time: 25 Minutes
Ingredients:
- 1 chopped green bell pepper, seeded
- 4 bacon slices
- ½ c. Parmesan Cheese
- 1 tbsp. avocado mayonnaise
- 2 chopped scallions

Directions:
1. Arrange bacon slices in the pot of Ninja Foodi and top with avocado mayonnaise, bell peppers, scallions and Parmesan Cheese.
2. Press "Bake/Roast" and set the timer to 25 minutes at 365 degrees F.
3. Remove from the Ninja Foodi after 25 minutes and dish out to serve.

- **Nutrition Info:** 197 calories, 13.8g fat, 4.7g carbs, 14.3g protein

20. Spinach Quiche

Servings: 6
Cooking Time: 45 Minutes
Ingredients:
- 1 tbsp. melted butter
- 10 oz. frozen and thawed spinach
- 5 beaten eggs
- Salt and black pepper
- 3 c. shredded Monterey Jack cheese

Directions:
1. Press "Sauté" on Ninja Foodi and add butter and spinach.
2. Sauté for about 3 minutes and dish out in a bowl.
3. Add eggs, Monterey Jack cheese, salt and black pepper to a bowl and transfer into greased molds.
4. Place the molds inside the pot of Ninja Foodi and press "Bake/Roast".
5. Set the timer to 30 minutes at 360 degrees F and press "Start".
6. Remove from the Ninja Foodi after 30 minutes and cut into equal sized wedges to serve.
- **Nutrition Info:** 349 calories, 27.8g fat, 3.2g carbs, 23g protein

21. Sausage And Spinach Breakfast Casserole

Servings: 6 -8 Servings
Cooking Time: 6 – 8 Hours
Ingredients:
- 1 pound breakfast sausage, casings removed
- 5 cups baby spinach, packed
- 1 bag of O'Brien potatoes, frozen
- 2 cups milk
- 8 eggs
- 1 ¼ cups Swiss cheese, grated
- 1 small onion, chopped fine
- ¼ cup Parmesan cheese, grated
- 2 teaspoons Dijon mustard
- 1 ½ teaspoons oregano
- 1 ½ teaspoons salt
- ¼ teaspoon freshly ground black pepper

- Red pepper flakes or hot sauce, for serving

Directions:
1. Set cooker to sauté on med-high heat. Add sausage, onion, and oregano and cook, breaking up the sausage till no longer pink, about 8 minutes. Add spinach and stir till wilted. Drain off the excess fat.
2. Add potatoes, 1 cup Swiss cheese, and the Parmesan cheese and stir to combine.
3. In a large bowl, whisk eggs, milk, mustard, salt and pepper together. Pour over sausage mix making sure you have an even layer.
4. Secure the lid and select slow cooker function on low heat. Cook 6 -8 hours or till the eggs are set. Top with remaining Swiss cheese and replace lid till it melts. Serve with pepper flakes or hot sauce if you like.

22. Avocado Eggs

Servings: 4
Cooking Time: 7 Minutes
Ingredients:
- 4 eggs
- 2 Avocados, sliced
- ¼ tsp salt
- ¼ tsp ground black pepper

Directions:
1. Prepare a baking pan that fits in your Ninja Foodi bowl by greasing the pan with butter. Set aside
2. Crack the eggs into the prepared baking pan and sprinkle with the salt and pepper. Lower the pan into the Ninja Foodi.
3. Set the Ninja Foodi to air crisp at 325 for 7 minutes.
4. Remove the pan of eggs from the Ninja Foodi and place the sliced avocado on top. Enjoy while hot!
- **Nutrition Info:** Calories: 190g, Carbohydrates: 7g , Protein: 8g, Fat: 15g, Sugar: 2g, Sodium: 657 g

23. French Toast & Cream Cheese Casserole

Servings: 4 - 6 Servings
Cooking Time: 45 Minutes
Ingredients:

- 1 small loaf of bread, sourdough or challah is ideal
- 1 cup milk
- 4 eggs
- ½ cup cream cheese, soft
- ½ cup brown sugar, packed
- 1 tablespoon powdered sugar
- 1 ½ teaspoons vanilla, divided
- ½ teaspoon cinnamon
- Streusel Topping
- ¼ cup brown sugar
- ¼ cup flour
- 3 tablespoons butter, cold and cubed
- ½ teaspoon cinnamon

Directions:
1. Lightly spray cooking pot with cooking spray.
2. Slice the bread then cut it into 1-inch cubed. Layer half of them in the prepared cooking pot.
3. In a mixing bowl, beat the cream cheese till smooth. Add powdered sugar and ¼ teaspoon of the vanilla and mix till combined. Drop by spoonful's on top of the bread. Add remaining bread cubes.
4. In a separate bowl, whisk together eggs, milk, cinnamon, brown sugar and remaining vanilla till combined and no lumps remain. Pour over the bread. Cover tightly with plastic wrap and refrigerate 3 hours or overnight.
5. Before baking, remove from refrigerator and prepare the topping: In a small bowl, stir together the dry ingredients. Cut in butter with a pastry knife or two forks. Sprinkle over the bread mixture.
6. Place the pot in the cooker and secure the Tender Crisp lid. Set the temperature to 350 degrees and bake for 45 minutes or golden brown on top. Serve it while warm with fruit or syrup.

24. Bacon, Tomato And Eggs

Servings: 4
Cooking Time: 7 Minutes
Ingredients:
- 4 eggs
- 1 Tbsp milk
- ½ cup crumbled bacon
- 1 tomato, diced
- ¼ tsp salt
- ¼ tsp ground black pepper

Directions:
1. Prepare a baking pan that fits in your Ninja Foodi bowl by greasing the pan with butter. Set aside
2. In a medium bowl, whisk together the eggs, milk, salt and pepper and then add the ham and cheese to the bowl and stir briefly.
3. Pour the egg mix into the prepared baking pan and lower the pan into the Ninja Foodi.
4. Set the Ninja Foodi to air crisp at 325 for 7 minutes.
5. Remove the pan of eggs from the Ninja Foodi and enjoy while hot!
- **Nutrition Info:** Calories: 157g, Carbohydrates: 2g , Protein: 11g, Fat: 12g, Sugar: 3g, Sodium: 957 g

25. Three Cheese Eggs

Servings: 4
Cooking Time: 7 Minutes
Ingredients:
- 4 eggs
- 1 Tbsp milk
- ¼ cup Shredded cheddar cheese
- ¼ cup swiss cheese
- ¼ cup American cheese
- ¼ tsp salt
- ¼ tsp ground black pepper

Directions:
1. Prepare a baking pan that fits in your Ninja Foodi bowl by greasing the pan with butter. Set aside
2. In a medium bowl, whisk together the eggs, milk, salt and pepper and then add the ham and cheese to the bowl and stir briefly.
3. Pour the egg mix into the prepared baking pan and lower the pan into the Ninja Foodi.
4. Set the Ninja Foodi to air crisp at 325 for 7 minutes.
5. Remove the pan of eggs from the Ninja Foodi and enjoy while hot!
- **Nutrition Info:** Calories: 138g, Carbohydrates: 1g , Protein: 11g, Fat: 10g, Sugar: 2g, Sodium: 711 g

26. Maple Sausage Bread Pudding

Servings: 4 -6 Servings
Cooking Time: 7 -8 Hours
Ingredients:

- 1 pound sausage, casings removed
- 1 small baguette, cubed
- 2 cups milk
- 1 ½ cups cheddar cheese, cubed
- ½ cup heavy cream
- ½ cup maple syrup
- 4 eggs

Directions:

1. Set cooker to sauté on med heat and add sausage. Cook, breaking it up into bite-size pieces, do not crumble it. Transfer to strainer and drain off fat. Cool completely.
2. In a large mixing bowl, whisk together eggs, milk, cream and syrup till smooth. Add the bread pieces, sausage and cheese and stir to combine, most of the liquid should soak into the bread.
3. Set the cooker to slow cooking function on low heat. Secure the lid and cook 7 -8 hours, or overnight. Serve warm drizzled with more maple syrup.

27. Walnut Date Oatmeal

Servings: 2 -3 Servings
Cooking Time: 3 Minutes
Ingredients:

- 2 ¼ cups water
- 1 cup old-fashioned rolled oats
- 2 tablespoons walnuts, chopped
- 2 tablespoons dates, pitted and chopped
- ½ banana, sliced

Directions:

1. Add all ingredients to the cooking pot.
2. Secure lid and select pressure cooker setting with high pressure. Set timer for 3 minutes. When timer goes off use quick release to remove the lid. Stir and serve drizzled with honey or brown sugar.

28. Baked Biscuits & Gravy

Servings: 4 Servings
Cooking Time: 1 Hour
Ingredients:

- 1 tube refrigerated biscuits
- 1 pound sausage, cooked and drained
- 4 eggs
- 1 cup cheddar cheese, grated
- 1/3 cup milk
- ½ teaspoon pepper
- ½ teaspoon salt
- For the gravy
- 2 cups milk
- 4 tablespoons butter
- 4 tablespoons flour
- ½ teaspoon salt
- ½ teaspoon pepper

Directions:

1. Cut each biscuit into 8 pieces. Set aside.
2. Mix the eggs, milk, salt and pepper in a bowl till combined.
3. Set the cooker to sauté on medium heat. Add butter and melt. Stir in flour, salt and pepper and while stirring, slowly pour in the milk.
4. Increase the heat to med-high and simmer gravy till it thickens. Transfer to a small bowl.
5. Wipe out the inside of the cooker and spray it lightly with cooking spray.
6. Add biscuit pieces to the cooker, then add sausage, cheese, egg mix and top with gravy.
7. Lock the Tender Crisp lid in place and set the temperature to 350 degrees. Bake for 35 – 45 minutes or eggs are cooked through.

29. Tofu With Mushrooms

Servings: 6
Cooking Time: 10 Minutes
Ingredients:

- 8 tbsps. shredded Parmesan cheese
- 2 c. freshly chopped mushrooms
- 2 blocks tofu, cubed
- Salt and black pepper
- 8 tbsps. butter

Directions:

1. Mix together tofu, salt and black pepper in a bowl.
2. Press "Sauté" on Ninja Foodi and add butter and seasoned tofu.
3. Sauté for about 5 minutes and add mushrooms and Parmesan cheese.

4. Sauté for about 3 minutes and press "Air Crisp".
5. Cook for about 2 minutes at 350 degrees F and dish out in a serving plate.
- **Nutrition Info:** 211 calories, 18.5g fat, 2g carbs, 11.5g protein

30. Eggs Benedict Bread Pudding

Servings: 4 – 6 Servings
Cooking Time: 90 Minutes
Ingredients:
- ½ pound Canadian bacon, cubed
- 4 asparagus spears, ends trimmed and cut into ½ inch pieces
- 3 English muffins, separated and cut into quarters
- 1 ½ cups milk
- 1 ½ cups half-and-half
- 6 eggs
- 1 package Hollandaise sauce mix
- 2 tablespoons fresh chives, chopped fine
- 1 teaspoon salt
- ¾ teaspoon white pepper
- For the Hollandaise Sauce
- ¾ cup butter, cubed
- 3 large egg yolks
- 1 ½ teaspoons fresh lemon juice
- ½ teaspoon salt
- Pinch of white pepper
- Pinch of cayenne

Directions:
1. Make the main part of the dish the night before serving. Heat oven to 375 degrees.
2. Place muffin pieces on a baking sheet and cook for 10 – 12 minutes or till toasted and crunchy.
3. Set the cooker to sauté on med-high heat. Add bacon and cook till lightly browned. Add in asparagus and cook, stirring often, about 4 minutes. Add toasted muffin pieces to bacon mix and toss well.
4. In a large mixing bowl, whisk together sauce mix packet and milk. Add eggs, half-and-half, salt, and pepper and whisk till thoroughly combined. Add the bacon mixture and stir well. Cover with foil and refrigerate 6 hours or overnight.
5. In the morning, remove the pudding mix from the fridge and let come to room temperature.
6. Lightly spray the cooking pot with cooking spray and attach the Tender Crisp lid. Transfer the egg mixture to the cooking pot and top with chives. Secure the lid and set temperature to 350 degrees. Bake for 45 minutes or it passes the toothpick test.
7. While it is baking prepare the Hollandaise sauce: place the butter in a saucepan over medium heat and melt till frothy, but not boiling.
8. Place remaining ingredients in a blender and process till combined. Keep the blender running as you slowly add the melted butter. The sauce will thicken, it is best to make the sauce during the last 10 minutes of baking time.
9. To serve, cut the bread pudding into wedges and top with the sauce. Enjoy.

31. Veggie Egg Casserole

Servings: 4
Cooking Time: 7 Minutes
Ingredients:
- 4 eggs
- 1 Tbsp milk
- 1 tomato, diced
- ½ cup spinach
- ¼ tsp salt
- ¼ tsp ground black pepper

Directions:
1. Prepare a baking pan that fits in your Ninja Foodi bowl by greasing the pan with butter. Set aside
2. In a medium bowl, whisk together the eggs, milk, salt and pepper and then add the veggies to the bowl and stir briefly.
3. Pour the egg mix into the prepared baking pan and lower the pan into the Ninja Foodi.
4. Set the Ninja Foodi to air crisp at 325 for 7 minutes.
5. Remove the pan of eggs from the Ninja Foodi and enjoy while hot!
- **Nutrition Info:** Calories: 78g, Carbohydrates: 1g , Protein: 7g, Fat: 5g, Sugar: 2g, Sodium: 660 g

32. Sweet And Savory Oatmeal

Servings: 6
Cooking Time: 10 Minutes
Ingredients:

- 3 cups almond milk
- 2 cups water
- ½ cup psyllium husks
- 1 ½ tsp vanilla extract
- ½ tsp cinnamon
- ¼ tsp nutmeg
- ½ cup granulated stevia
- ½ cup crumbled, cooked bacon

Directions:

1. Add all of the ingredients into the Ninja Foodi and stir together briefly
2. Place the lid on and set the steamer valve to seal. Set the pressure cooker function to 1 minute (it will take about 10 minutes to come to pressure).
3. When the oatmeal is done, do a quick pressure release by opening the steamer valve carefully. Serve while hot
- **Nutrition Info:** Calories: 65g, Carbohydrates: 4g , Protein: 1g, Fat: 8g, Sugar: 0g, Sodium: 316 g

33. Mini Frittatas

Servings: 5
Cooking Time: 10 Minutes
Ingredients:

- 5 eggs
- Splash of almond milk
- Salt and pepper
- Desired mix in's: cheese, veggies, meats, the options are endless!

Directions:

1. Preparing the ingredients, Mix eggs, milk, and mix-in's in a dish. Pour mixture into individual baking molds. Place molds on rack in Ninja Foodi with 1 cup of water.
2. High pressure for 5 minutes. Close the lid and the pressure valve and then cook for 5 minutes. To get 5-minutes cook time, press "Pressure" button and use the TIME ADJUSTMENT button to adjust the cook time to 5 minutes.

3. Pressure Release Use the quick-release method when the timer goes off and cooking is done.
4. Enjoy!
- **Nutrition Info:** 342.5 calories, 23.7g fat, 8.2g carbs, 25g protein

34. Caramel Pumpkin Oatmeal

Servings: 10 Servings
Cooking Time: 2 Hours
Ingredients:

- 5 -7 cups milk
- 2 cups rolled oats
- ½ cup pumpkin
- ½ cup date paste
- 2 teaspoon cinnamon
- ½ teaspoon ginger
- ¼ teaspoon nutmeg

Directions:

1. Add all ingredients to the cooking pot. Secure the lid and select slow cooker function on high heat. Set timer for 2 hours.
2. Stir before serving. Store any left overs in an airtight container in the refrigerator.

35. Almond French Toast Bites

Servings: 3 Serving
Cooking Time: 15 Minutes
Ingredients:

- 8 pieces of bread
- 6 eggs
- 1/3 cup sugar
- 2 tablespoons almond milk
- 2 tablespoons cinnamon

Directions:

1. Whisk the eggs and almond milk together in a small bowl.
2. In a separate small bowl mix the sugar and cinnamon together.
3. Tear the bread in half and roll the halves into balls, pressing them firmly together.
4. Soak the balls in the egg till it starts to soak into the bread, then roll them in the cinnamon sugar.
5. Place the balls, 8 at a time, in the basket for the air fryer. Lock the Tender Crisp lid in place and set the temperature to 360

degrees. Cook the bites 15 minutes, or till they are crisp.

6. Serve them with maple syrup for dipping or eat them as they are.

36. Raspberry Breakfast Cake

Servings: 6
Cooking Time: 25 Minutes
Ingredients:

- 8 Tbsp butter
- ½ cup Baking Stevia
- 1 egg
- 1 tsp vanilla
- 2 cups almond flour
- 2 tsp baking powder
- 1 tsp salt
- 1 cup fresh raspberries
- ½ cup buttermilk

Directions:

1. Use an electric mixer to cream the butter and stevia together until they are light and fluffy.
2. Mix the vanilla and eggs in a small bowl then add to the mixer with the butter blend. Ix until just combined
3. In a separate bowl, toss the raspberries and ¼ cup almond flour to coat the berries.
4. Add the remaining dry ingredients to the mixer and fold together by hand. Add the buttermilk and mix until smooth.
5. Add the raspberries to the batter and mix briefly.
6. Pour the cake batter into your Ninja Foodi and place the lid on.
7. Press the air crisp button and set the temperature to 350 degrees and program the timer to 25 minutes.
8. Once cooked, a toothpick should come out of the center of the cake cleanly. Allow to cool and serve.
- **Nutrition Info:** Calories: 183 g, Carbohydrates: 8g, Protein: 3g, Fat: 16 g, Sugar: 3g, Sodium: 464 g

37. Bacon, Broccoli And Cheddar Frittata

Servings: 4
Cooking Time: 7 Minutes
Ingredients:

- 6 eggs
- 2 Tbsp milk
- ½ cup chopped, cooked bacon
- 1 cup cooked broccoli
- ½ cup shredded cheddar cheese
- ¼ tsp salt
- ¼ tsp ground black pepper

Directions:

1. Prepare a baking pan that fits in your Ninja Foodi bowl by greasing the pan with butter. Set aside
2. In a medium bowl, whisk together the eggs, milk, salt and pepper and then add the bacon, broccoli and cheese to the bowl and stir briefly.
3. Pour the egg mix into the prepared baking pan and lower the pan into the Ninja Foodi.
4. Set the Ninja Foodi to air crisp at 325 for 7 minutes.
5. Remove the pan of eggs from the Ninja Foodi and enjoy while hot!
- **Nutrition Info:** Calories: 269g, Carbohydrates: 3g, Protein: 19g, Fat: 20g, Sugar: 2g, Sodium: 370 g

38. Pepperoni Omelet

Servings: 4
Cooking Time: 5 Minutes
Ingredients:

- 4 tbsps. heavy cream
- 15 pepperoni slices
- 2 tbsps. butter
- Salt and black pepper
- 6 eggs

Directions:

1. Whisk together the eggs, heavy cream, pepperoni slices, salt and black pepper in a bowl.
2. Press "Sauté" on Ninja Foodi and add butter and egg mixture.
3. Sauté for about 3 minutes and flip the side of the omelette.
4. Lock the lid and set the Ninja Foodi on "Air Crisp" for about 2 minutes at 350 degrees F.
5. Dish out in a serving plate and serve with low carb bread.
- **Nutrition Info:** 141 calories, 11.3g fat, 0.6g carbs, 8.9g protein

39. Ham And Eggs Casserole

Servings: 4

Cooking Time: 7 Minutes

Ingredients:

- 4 eggs
- 1 Tbsp milk
- 1 cup cooked, chopped ham
- ½ cup Shredded cheddar cheese
- ¼ tsp salt
- ¼ tsp ground black pepper

Directions:

1. Prepare a baking pan that fits in your Ninja Foodi bowl by greasing the pan with butter. Set aside
2. In a medium bowl, whisk together the eggs, milk, salt and pepper and then add the ham and cheese to the bowl and stir briefly.
3. Pour the egg mix into the prepared baking pan and lower the pan into the Ninja Foodi.
4. Set the Ninja Foodi to air crisp at 325 for 7 minutes.
5. Remove the pan of eggs from the Ninja Foodi and enjoy while hot!

- **Nutrition Info:** Calories: 169g, Carbohydrates: 1g , Protein: 12g, Fat: 13g, Sugar: 1g, Sodium: 455 g

40. Ham Spinach Ballet

Servings: 8

Cooking Time: 35 Minutes

Ingredients:

- 3 lbs. fresh baby spinach
- ½ c. cream
- 28 oz. sliced ham
- 4 tbsps. melted butter
- Salt and freshly ground black pepper

Directions:

1. Press "Sauté" on Ninja Foodi and add butter and spinach.
2. Sauté for about 3 minutes and top with cream, ham slices, salt and black pepper.
3. Lock the lid and set the Ninja Foodi to "Bake/Roast" for about 8 minutes at 360 degrees F.
4. Remove from the Ninja Foodi after 8 minutes and dish out to serve.

- **Nutrition Info:** 188 calories, 12.5g fat, 4.9g carbs, 14.6g protein

MEAT RECIPES

41. Chili Chicken Wings

Servings: 4 Servings
Cooking Time: 28 Minutes
Ingredients:
- ½ cup water
- ½ cup hot sauce
- 2 Tbsp butter
- 1 ½ tbsp. apple cider vinegar
- 32 ounces frozen chicken wings
- ½ tsp paprika

Directions:
1. Add all the ingredients into the cook and crisp basket and place the basket inside the Ninja Foodi.
2. Place the pressure cooker lid on top of the pot and close the pressure valve to the seal position. Set the pressure cooker function to high heat and set the timer for 5 minutes.
3. Once the coking cycle is complete, release the pressure quickly by carefully opening the steamer valve. Enjoy while hot
- **Nutrition Info:** Calories: 311g , Carbohydrates: 0g, Protein: 24g, Fat: 23g, Sugar: 0g, Sodium: 2657 mg

42. Healthy 'n Tasty Meatloaf

Servings: 2
Cooking Time: 20 Minutes
Ingredients:
- 3/4-pound ground beef
- 3/4 cup bread crumbs
- 1/3 cup parmesan cheese
- 2 small eggs, beaten
- 1 tablespoon minced garlic
- 1 teaspoon steak seasoning
- Salt and pepper to taste
- 1 1/2 teaspoons sear button sugar
- 1/4 cup ketchup
- 1/2 tablespoon mustard
- 1 teaspoon Worcestershire sauce

Directions:
1. Place a trivet in the Ninja Foodi and pour a cup of beef broth.
2. In a mixing bowl, mix together the beef, bread crumbs, cheese, eggs, garlic, and steak seasoning. Season with salt and pepper to taste.
3. Pour meat mixture in a heat-proof pan and place on top of the trivet. Cover top with foil.
4. Install pressure lid. Close Ninja Foodi, press the steam button, and set time to 20 minutes.
5. While waiting for the meatloaf to cook, combine in a saucepan the sugar, ketchup, mustard, and Worcestershire sauce. Mix until the sauce becomes thick.
6. Once done cooking, do a quick release.
7. Remove the meatloaf from the Ninja Foodi and allow to cool.
8. Serve with sauce and enjoy.
- **Nutrition Info:** Calories: 574; carbohydrates: 23.2g; protein: 46.6g; fat: 32.7g

43. Indian Keema Matar Chicken

Servings: 2
Cooking Time: 25 Minutes
Ingredients:
- 2 tablespoons oil
- 1 tablespoon garlic paste
- 1 tablespoon ginger paste
- 1 onion, chopped
- 1-pound ground chicken
- 2 teaspoon coriander powder
- 1 teaspoon cayenne pepper
- 1 teaspoon garam masala
- ½ teaspoon ground cumin
- Salt and pepper to taste
- 2 tomatoes, diced
- ½ cup green peas
- ¼ cup water
- 1 tablespoon lemon juice
- ½ cup mint leaves

Directions:
1. Press the sauté button on the Ninja Foodi and heat the oil and sauté the garlic and ginger paste. Add the onion and sauté until fragrant.
2. Stir the chicken and season with coriander powder, cayenne pepper, garam masala,

and cumin. Season with salt and pepper to taste. Stir for 3 minutes.
3. Add the tomato, green peas, water, and lemon juice.
4. Install pressure lid. Close Ninja Foodi, press the manual button, choose high settings, and set time to 20 minutes.
5. Once done cooking, do a quick release. Garnish with chopped mint leaves.
6. Serve and enjoy.
- **Nutrition Info:** Calories: 560; carbohydrates:20.7g; protein: 44.8g; fat: 33.1g

44. Beef ' N Mushrooms In Thick Sauce

Servings: 2
Cooking Time: 35 Minutes
Ingredients:
- 1/2 tablespoon butter
- 1/2-pound beef chunks
- Salt and pepper to taste
- 1/2 cup onions, chopped
- 1/2 tablespoon garlic, minced
- 1 carrot, sliced diagonally
- 1/4 cup chopped celery
- 1/3 cup mushrooms, halved
- 1 medium potato, peeled and quartered
- 1 tablespoon Worcestershire sauce
- 1 tablespoon tomato paste
- 1/2 cup chicken broth
- 1 tablespoon all-purpose flour + 1 tablespoon water

Directions:
1. Turn on the sauté button on the Ninja Foodi and melt the butter. Sear button the beef chunks and season with salt and pepper to taste. Add the onions and garlic until fragrant.
2. Stir in the carrots, celery, mushrooms and potatoes.
3. Add the Worcestershire sauce, tomato paste, and chicken broth. Season with more salt and pepper to taste.
4. Install pressure lid. Close Ninja Foodi, press the pressure button, choose high settings, and set time to 30 minutes.
5. Once done cooking, do a quick release.

6. Open the lid and press the sauté button. Stir in the all-purpose flour and allow to simmer until the sauce thickens.
7. Serve and enjoy.
- **Nutrition Info:** Calories: 539; carbohydrates: 61.3g; protein:43.9g; fat: 13.1g

45. Chicken Alfredo Pasta

Servings: 3
Cooking Time: 5 Minutes
Ingredients:
- 8 oz. fettuccine
- 15 oz. Alfredo sauce
- 2 c. water
- 1 c. cooked chicken, diced
- 2 tsps. chicken seasoning

Directions:
1. Break your pasta in half so it fits in the cooker.
2. Add pasta, water, and chicken seasoning to Ninja Foodi.
3. Seal the lid. Select STEAM and cook at HIGH pressure for 3 minutes.
4. When the timer beeps, press CANCEL and use a quick release.
5. Drain the pasta and add to serving bowl.
6. Mix in Alfredo sauce and chicken. Serve!
- **Nutrition Info:** 225 calories, 6.3g fat, 21.8g carbs, 20.1g protein

46. Tasty Sesame-honeyed Chicken

Servings: 2
Cooking Time: 16 Minutes
Ingredients:
- 1 tablespoon olive oil
- 1/2 onion, diced
- 2 cloves of garlic, minced
- 1-pound chicken breasts
- 1/4 cup soy sauce
- 2 tbsp ketchup
- 1 tsp sesame oil
- 1/4 cup honey
- ½ teaspoon red pepper flakes
- 1 tablespoon cornstarch + 1 1/2 tablespoons water
- Green onions for garnish
- 1 tablespoon sesame seeds for garnish

Directions:

1. Press the sauté button on the Ninja Foodi and heat the oil. Stir in the onion and garlic until fragrant.
2. Add the chicken breasts. Allow to sear on all sides for three minutes.
3. Stir in the soy sauce, ketchup, sesame oil, honey, and red pepper flakes.
4. Install pressure lid. Close Ninja Foodi, press the pressure button, choose high settings, and set time to 10 minutes.
5. Once done cooking, do a quick release.
6. Open the lid and press the sauté button. Stir in the cornstarch slurry and allow to simmer until the sauce thickens.
7. Garnish with green onions and sesame seeds last.
8. Serve and enjoy.
- **Nutrition Info:** Calories: 568; carbohydrates: 49.1g; protein: 50.9g; fat: 34.6g

47. Chicken Shawarma Middle-east

Servings: 2
Cooking Time: 20 Minutes
Ingredients:

- ¼ teaspoon coriander
- ¼ teaspoon cumin
- ½ teaspoon paprika
- 1 teaspoon cardamom
- ½ teaspoon cinnamon powder
- ¼ teaspoon cloves
- ¼ teaspoon nutmeg
- ¼ cup lemon juice
- ¼ cup yogurt
- 2 tablespoons garlic, minced
- 1-pound boneless chicken breasts, cut into strips
- 2 bay leaves
- Salt and pepper to taste
- 2 pita bread
- ¼ cup greek yogurt
- For garnish: tomatoes, lettuce, and cucumber

Directions:

1. Place in the Ninja Foodi the coriander, cumin, paprika, cardamom, cinnamon powder, cloves, nutmeg, lemon juice, yogurt, garlic, and chicken breasts. Add the bay leaves and season with salt and pepper to taste.
2. Install pressure lid. Close Ninja Foodi, press the pressure button, choose high settings, and set time to 20 minutes.
3. Once done cooking, do a quick release. Place the chicken in the pita bread and drizzle with Greek yogurt. Garnish with tomatoes, lettuce, and cucumber.
4. Serve and enjoy.
- **Nutrition Info:** Calories: 372; carbohydrates: 21.8g; protein: 55.1g; fat: 7.1g

48. Slow Cooking Beef Fajitas

Servings: 8
Cooking Time: 7 Hours 8 Minutes
Ingredients:

- 2 tbsps. butter
- 2 sliced bell peppers
- 2 lbs. sliced beef
- 2 tbsps. fajita seasoning
- 2 sliced onions

Directions:

1. Press "Sauté" on Ninja Foodi and add butter, onions, fajita seasoning, bell pepper and beef.
2. Sauté for about 3 minutes and press "Slow Cooker".
3. Cook for 7 hours on Low and dish out to serve hot.
- **Nutrition Info:** 353 calories, 13.4g fat, 8.5g carbs, 46.7g protein

49. Roasted Crisp Whole Chicken

Servings: 2
Cooking Time: 25 Minutes
Ingredients:

- 1 whole Cornish Hen
- 1/2 tsp seasoned salt
- Juice of 1/2 lemon
- 1 tbsp honey
- ¼ cup hot water
- 1/4 teaspoon salt
- 1/2 teaspoon whole peppercorns (optional)
- 1 sprigs of fresh thyme
- 2 cloves of garlic

- 1 tsp canola oil

Directions:

1. Combine lemon juice, honey, water, salt, peppercorns, thyme, and garlic in pot.
2. Season the chicken inside, outside and underneath the skin with seasoned salt.
3. Place the chicken in the air crisp basket then place into the pot.
4. Install pressure lid. Close pot, choose high, and cook for 15 minutes.
5. Once done cooking, do a quick release. Remove pressure lid.
6. Brush the chicken with canola oil
7. Close the crisping lid and select roast.
8. Set the time for 15 minutes and halfway through cooking time turn chicken over.
9. The juices in the bottom of the cooking pot make a delicious sauce.
- **Nutrition Info:** Calories: 196; carbohydrates: 10.5g; protein: 24.2g; fat: 6.3g

50. Crispy Garlic-parmesan Wings

Servings: 2
Cooking Time: 20 Minutes
Ingredients:

- 1-lb chicken wings/drumettes
- Seasoned salt, to season the wings
- 1/2 cup of chicken broth
- Sauce Ingredients:
- 1 stick of salted butter, melted
- 1/2 tsp of garlic better than bouillon (or 1 tbsp of crushed garlic)
- 1/2 cup of grated parmesan cheese
- 1 tsp of garlic powder
- 1/2 tsp of black pepper
- 1/2 tsp of dried parsley flakes

Directions:

1. Lightly rub the seasoned salt on both sides of the chicken wings
2. Add the wings to the Ninja Foodi followed by the broth.
3. Install pressure lid. Close Ninja Foodi, press pressure button, select high settings, and cook for 8 minutes.
4. While the wings are pressure cooking, make the garlic parmesan sauce by combining the butter, garlic, parmesan, pepper, garlic

powder and parsley flakes in a large bowl. Mix together well.

5. Once the wings are done cooking, do a quick release.
6. Transfer to bowl of sauce and discard liquid. Remove pressure lid.
7. Add the trivet to pot, spray with non-stick spray and place wings.
8. Lower the tendercrisp lid and hit "broil" and go for 8-10 minutes (the longer you go, the crispier the wings so be sure to check on them). It is a good idea to flip the wings midway through the crisping process.
9. Enjoy!
- **Nutrition Info:** Calories: 957; carbohydrates: 5.5g; protein: 63.0g; fat: 75.9g

51. Chicken Congee

Servings: 7
Cooking Time: 65 Minutes
Ingredients:

- 6 chicken drumsticks
- 7 c. water
- 1 c. Jasmine rice
- 1 tbsp. ginger, fresh
- Salt

Directions:

1. Rinse rice under cool water for a few minutes.
2. Pour rice, water, ginger, and drumsticks into Ninja Foodi. Seal the lid.
3. Select "PRESSURE" and cook at HIGH pressure for 30 minutes.
4. When time is up, press CANCEL and wait for a natural pressure release.
5. When safe, open the lid and press "SAUTÉ".
6. Keep stirring while the congee thickens.
7. Season with salt.
8. Pull off the chicken with tongs, and throw away the bones.
9. Serve right away!
- **Nutrition Info:** 181 calories, 6g fat, 21g carbs, 12g protein

52. Easy Kung Pao Chicken

Servings: 2
Cooking Time: 20 Minutes

Ingredients:
- 1 tablespoon olive oil
- 1 clove garlic, minced
- 1/2 teaspoon grated ginger
- 1/2 teaspoon crushed red pepper
- 1/2 onion, chopped
- 1-pound chicken breasts, cut into bite-sized pieces
- 1/4 cup soy sauce
- 2 tbsp honey
- 2 tbsp hoisin sauce
- 1/2 zucchini, diced
- 1/2 red bell pepper, chopped

Directions:
1. Press the sauté button on the Ninja Foodi and heat the oil. Sauté the garlic, ginger, red pepper, and onion until fragrant.
2. Add the chicken breasts and stir for 3 minutes until lightly golden.
3. Stir in the soy sauce, honey, and hoisin sauce.
4. Close Ninja Foodi, press bake button, set temperature to 350 ºF, and set time to 20 minutes. Halfway through cooking time, stir and continue cooking.
5. Open the lid and press the sauté button. Stir in the zucchini and bell pepper. Allow to simmer until the vegetables are cooked.
6. Serve and enjoy.
- **Nutrition Info:** Calories: 501; carbohydrates: 29.4g; protein: 40.7g; fat: 24.5g

53. Hk Mushroom Gravy Over Chops

Servings: 2
Cooking Time: 25 Minutes
Ingredients:
- 2 bone-in pork loin chops
- 1/2 onion, chopped
- 2 cloves of garlic, minced
- 10 large cremini mushrooms, sliced
- A dash of sherry wine
- 3/4 cup chicken stock
- 1 tablespoon Worcestershire sauce
- 1 tablespoon soy sauce
- 1 tablespoon peanut oil
- 2 tbsp heavy cream
- Salt and pepper to taste
- 1 tablespoon cornstarch + 1 tablespoon water

Directions:
1. Press the sauté button on the Ninja Foodi. Place the pork chops and sear on all sides for 5 minutes each. Stir in the onion and garlic until fragrant.
2. Add the mushrooms, sherry wine, chicken stock, Worcestershire sauce, soy sauce, peanut oil and cream. Season with salt and pepper to taste.
3. Install pressure lid. Close Ninja Foodi, press the pressure button, choose high settings, and set time to 20 minutes.
4. Once done cooking, do a quick release.
5. Once the lid is open, press the sauté button and stir in cornstarch slurry. Allow to simmer until the sauce thickens.
6. Serve and enjoy.
- **Nutrition Info:** Calories: 481; carbohydrates: 10.4g; protein: 44.6g; fat: 28.9g

54. Herbed Lamb Chops

Servings: 4
Cooking Time: 10 Hours
Ingredients:
- 1 lb. lamb chops
- 1½ C. tomatoes, chopped finely
- 1 C. chicken broth
- Salt and freshly ground black pepper, to taste
- 3 tbsp. mixed fresh herbs (oregano, thyme, sage), chopped

Directions:
1. In the pot of Ninja Foodi, place all the ingredients and mix well.
2. Close the crisping lid and select "Slow Cooker".
3. Set on "Low" for about 8 hours.
4. Press "Start/Stop" to begin.
5. Open the lid and serve hot.
- **Nutrition Info:** Calories: 237; Carbohydrates: 3.8g; Protein: 33.8g; Fat: 9g; Sugar: 2g; Sodium: 319mg; Fiber: 1.4g

55. Pulled Bbq Chicken

Servings: 6 Servings
Cooking Time: 15 Minutes
Ingredients:

- 1 ½ pounds boneless, skinless chicken thighs
- 1 Tbsp olive oil
- 1 tsp ground paprika
- ¼ tsp salt
- ¼ tsp ground black pepper
- 1 onion, chopped
- ¼ cup hot sauce
- ¼ cup water
- 2 Tbsp vinegar

Directions:

1. Turn the Ninja Foodi on to saute and add the olive oil. Once hot, add the chicken thighs and sear on each side for 2 minutes.
2. Sprinkle the salt and pepper on the chicken and then add all the remaining ingredients to the pot.
3. Cover the Foodi and use the pressure cooker function to cook the chicken for 15 minutes under high heat pressure.
4. Release the pressure using a natural steam release and then use two forks to pull he chicken apart. Serve warm or chilled
- **Nutrition Info:** Calories: 215g, Carbohydrates: 1g, Protein: 17g, Fat: 16g, Sugar: 1g, Sodium: 1672 mg

56. Smoky Roasted Chicken

Servings: 5
Cooking Time: 40 Minutes
Ingredients:

- 1 (4-lb.) whole chicken, necks and giblets removed
- Salt and freshly ground black pepper, to taste
- 1 tsp. liquid smoke
- 2 tbsp. chicken rub

Directions:

1. Season the chicken inside, outside and underneath the skin with the salt and black pepper generously.
2. In the pot of Ninja Foodi, place 1 C. of water and liquid smoke.

3. Place the chicken into the "Cook & Crisp Basket".
4. Arrange the "Cook & Crisp Basket" in the pot.
5. Cover the Ninja Foodi with the pressure lid and place the pressure valve to "Seal" position.
6. Select "Pressure" and set to "High" for about 15 minutes.
7. Press "Start/Stop" to begin.
8. Switch the valve to "Vent" and do a "Quick" release.
9. Once all the pressure is released, open the lid
10. Spray the chicken with the cooking spray and then, coat with half of the chicken rub.
11. Now, close the Ninja Foodi with the crisping lid and select "Air Crisp".
12. Set the temperature to 400 degrees F for 10 minutes.
13. Press "Start/Stop" to begin.
14. Again, spray the chicken with the cooking spray and then, coat with half of the chicken rub.
15. Close the Ninja Foodi with the crisping lid and cook for 10 minutes more.
16. Open the lid and transfer the chicken onto a cutting board for about 10 minutes before carving.
17. Cut into desired sized pieces and serve.
- **Nutrition Info:** Calories: 557; Carbohydrates: 1.2g; Protein: 3.2105.2g; Fat: 11g; Sugar: 0g; Sodium: 446mg; Fiber: 0g

57. Sweet & Sour Pork Chops

Servings: 4
Cooking Time: 16 Minutes
Ingredients:

- 6 pork loin chops
- Salt and freshly ground black pepper, to taste
- 2 tbsp. honey
- 2 tbsp. soy sauce
- 1 tbsp. balsamic vinegar

Directions:

1. With a meat tenderizer, tenderize the chops completely.

2. Sprinkle the chops with a little salt and black pepper.
3. In a large bowl, mix together remaining ingredients. Add the chops and coat with marinade generously. Refrigerate, covered for about 6-8 hours.
4. Arrange the "Cook & Crisp Basket" in the pot of Ninja Foodi. Close the Ninja Foodi with crisping lid and select "Air Crisp".
5. Press "Start/Stop" to begin and set the temperature to 355 degrees F.
6. Set the time for 5 minutes to preheat.
7. Now, place the pork chops into "Cook & Crisp Basket". Close the Ninja Foodi with crisping lid and select "Air Crisp". Set the temperature to 355 degrees F for 16 minutes, flipping once half way through.
8. Press "Start/Stop" to begin. Open the lid and serve hot.
- **Nutrition Info:** Calories: 281; Carbohydrates: 6.2g; Protein: 18.3g; Fat: 19.9g; Sugar: 5.9g; Sodium: 384mg; Fiber: 0.1g

58. Beef Chili

Servings: 4
Cooking Time: 8 Minutes
Ingredients:
- 1 pound beef roast
- 2 cups beef broth
- 2 cloves of garlic, chopped
- 1 bell pepper, chopped
- 1 white onion, chopped
- 4 tomatoes, chopped
- 1 tsp dried basil
- 1 tsp dried oregano
- ½ tsp tsp salt
- 1/8 tsp ground black pepper
- ¼ cup shredded cheddar cheese

Directions:
1. Place the beef roast in the Ninja Foodi pot and sprinkle with the oregano, salt, basil and ground black pepper.
2. Add the broth, garlic, tomato, bell pepper and onion to the pot and close the pressure cooker lid.
3. Cook on high pressure for 10 minutes. Do a quick steam release and remove the lid.

4. Add the cream cheese and heavy cream and stir to blend.
5. Sprinkle the cheese on top of the chili and put the air crisper top on. Use the broil function to brown the cheese for 2 minutes.
- **Nutrition Info:** Calories: 282g, Carbohydrates: 4g, Protein: 14g, Fat: 13g, Sugar: 2g , Sodium: 1163 mg

59. Jamaican Style Curried Chicken

Servings: 2
Cooking Time: 25 Minutes
Ingredients:
- 2 tablespoons oil
- 1 tablespoon minced garlic
- 1 cup chopped onion
- 1 ½ tablespoon jamaican curry powder
- 1 scotch bonnet pepper, sliced
- ½ teaspoon ground allspice
- 3 sprigs of thyme
- 1-pound boneless chicken thighs, chunked
- Salt and pepper to taste
- 1 large potato, cut into chunks
- 1 cup water

Directions:
1. Press the sauté button on the Ninja Foodi and sauté the garlic, onion, curry powder, scotch bonnet pepper, allspice, and thyme until fragrant.
2. Stir in the chicken thighs and cook until lightly golden. Season with salt and pepper to taste. Add the potatoes and water.
3. Install pressure lid and place valve to vent position.
4. Close Ninja Foodi, press the pressure button, choose high settings, and set time to 20 minutes.
5. Once done cooking, do a quick release. Serve and enjoy.
- **Nutrition Info:** Calories: 1099; carbohydrates: 78.5g; protein: 48.6g; fat: 65.6g

60. Jamaican Jerk Pork Roast

Servings: 3
Cooking Time: 33 Minutes
Ingredients:
- 1 tbsp. butter

- 1/8 c. beef broth
- 1 lb. pork shoulder
- 1/8 c. Jamaican jerk spice blend

Directions:
1. Season the pork with Jamaican jerk spice blend.
2. Press "Sauté" on Ninja Foodi and add butter and seasoned pork.
3. Sauté for about 3 minutes and add beef broth.
4. Press "Pressure" and cook for about 20 minutes on Low.
5. Release the pressure naturally and dish out in a platter.
- **Nutrition Info:** 477 calories, 36.2g fat, 2g carbs, 35.4g protein

61. Beef Stew Recipe From Ethiopia

Servings: 2
Cooking Time: 55 Minutes
Ingredients:
- 1-pound beef stew meat, cut into chunks
- ¼ teaspoon turmeric powder
- 1 tablespoon garam masala
- 1 tablespoon coriander powder
- 1 teaspoon cumin
- ¼ teaspoon ground nutmeg
- 2 teaspoons smoked paprika
- ¼ teaspoon black pepper
- 2 tablespoons ghee
- 1 onion, chopped
- 1 tablespoon ginger, grated
- 2 cloves of garlic, grated
- 1 tablespoon onions
- 3 tablespoons tomato paste
- ½ teaspoon sugar
- Salt and pepper to taste
- 1 cup water

Directions:
1. In a mixing bowl, combine the first 8 ingredients and allow to marinate in the fridge for at least 4 hours.
2. Press the sauté button and heat the oil. Sauté the onion, ginger, and garlic until fragrant. Stir in the marinated beef and allow to sear button for 3 minutes.
3. Stir in the rest of the ingredients.

4. Install pressure lid. Close Ninja Foodi, press the pressure button, choose high settings, and set time to 50 minutes.
5. Once done cooking, do a quick release.
6. Serve and enjoy.
- **Nutrition Info:** Calories: 591; carbohydrates: 11.5g; protein: 83.5g; fat: 23.4g

62. Bacon Swiss Pork Chops

Servings: 4
Cooking Time: 23 Minutes
Ingredients:
- ½ c. shredded Swiss cheese
- 4 pork chops
- 6 bacon strips, cut in half
- Salt and black pepper
- 1 tbsp. butter

Directions:
1. Apply black pepper and salt to the pork chops generously.
2. Press "Sauté" on Ninja Foodi and add butter and pork chops.
3. Sauté for about 3 minutes on each side and add bacon strips and Swiss cheese.
4. Press "Pressure" and set the timer to 15 minutes on Medium Low.
5. Transfer the steaks in a serving platter and serve hot.
- **Nutrition Info:** 483 calories, 40g fat, 0.7g carbs, 27.7g protein

63. Sweet And Sour Chicken Wings

Servings: 4 Servings
Cooking Time: 28 Minutes
Ingredients:
- ½ cup water
- 2 Tbsp baking stevia
- 2 Tbsp butter
- 2 Tbsp lemon juice
- 32 ounces frozen chicken wings
- ½ tsp salt
- ½ tsp ground black pepper

Directions:
1. Add all the ingredients into the cook and crisp basket and place the basket inside the Ninja Foodi.

2. Place the pressure cooker lid on top of the pot and close the pressure valve to the seal position. Set the pressure cooker function to high heat and set the timer for 5 minutes.
3. Once the coking cycle is complete, release the pressure quickly by carefully opening the steamer valve. Enjoy while hot
- **Nutrition Info:** Calories: 312g, Carbohydrates: 2g, Protein: 24g, Fat: 23g, Sugar: 2g, Sodium: 985 mg

64. Ranch Flavored Tender Wings

Servings: 2
Cooking Time: 20 Minutes
Ingredients:
- 1/2 cup water
- 1/4 cup hot pepper sauce
- 2 tablespoons unsalted butter, melted
- 1/2 tablespoons apple cider vinegar
- 1-pound chicken wings
- 1/4 (1-ounce) envelope ranch salad dressing mix
- 1/2 teaspoon paprika
- Nonstick cooking spray

Directions:
1. Pour the water, hot pepper sauce, butter, and vinegar into the pot. Place the wings in the cook & crisp basket and place the basket in the pot.
2. Install pressure lid. Close pot, press pressure button, select high settings, and cook for 5 minutes.
3. Once done, do a quick release. Remove pressure lid.
4. Sprinkle the chicken wings with the dressing mix and paprika. Coat with cooking spray.
5. Close Ninja Foodi, press air crisp, set the temperature to 375 ºF, and crisp for 15 minutes. Halfway through cooking time, turnover wings.
6. Serve and enjoy.
- **Nutrition Info:** Calories: 351; carbohydrates: 1.3g; protein: 50.5g; fat: 16.0g

65. Deliciously Spicy Turkey Legs

Servings: 2

Cooking Time: 25 Minutes
Ingredients:
- 2 turkey legs
- 5 C. chicken broth
- 3 tbsp. olive oil
- 1-2 tbsp. Mrs. Dash seasoning
- 1 tsp. paprika

Directions:
1. In the pot of Ninja Foodi, place turkey legs and top with the broth.
2. Cover the Ninja Foodi with the pressure lid and place the pressure valve to "Seal" position.
3. Select "Pressure" and set to "High" for about 15 minutes. Press "Start/Stop" to begin. Switch the valve to "Vent" and do a "Quick" release.
4. Once all the pressure is released, open the lid
5. Transfer the turkey legs onto a plate and with paper towels, pat dry them.
6. Remove broth from the pot and arrange the reversible rack in the pot.
7. Drizzle the turkey legs with oil and rub with the Mrs. Dash seasoning and paprika.
8. Place the turkey legs over the rack. Close the Ninja Foodi with the crisping lid and Select "Air Crisp". Set the temperature to 400 degrees F for 10 minutes.
9. Press "Start/Stop" to begin. After 7 minutes, flip the turkey legs.
10. Open the lid and serve.
- **Nutrition Info:** Calories: 634; Carbohydrates: 2.9g; Protein: 79.2g; Fat: 32.4g; Sugar: 1.9g; Sodium: 800mg; Fiber: 0.4g

66. Savory 'n Aromatic Chicken Adobo

Servings: 2
Cooking Time: 20 Minutes
Ingredients:
- 1-pound boneless chicken thighs
- 1/4 cup white vinegar
- ½ cup water
- 1/4 cup soy sauce
- 1/2 head garlic, peeled and smashed
- 2 bay leaves
- ½ teaspoon pepper

- 1 tsp oil

Directions:
1. Place all ingredients in the Ninja Foodi.
2. Install pressure lid. Close Ninja Foodi, press the pressure button, choose high settings, and set time to 10 minutes.
3. Once done cooking, do a quick release.
4. Open the lid and press the sauté button. Allow the sauce to reduce so that the chicken is fried slightly in its oil, around 10 minutes.
5. Serve and enjoy.
- **Nutrition Info:** Calories: 713; carbohydrates: 3.2g; protein: 43.9g; fat: 58.3g

67. Yummy Turkey Tenderloins

Servings: 6
Cooking Time: 23 Minutes
Ingredients:
- 1 tsp. dried thyme, crushed
- 1 tsp. garlic powder
- Salt and freshly ground black pepper, to taste
- 1 (24-oz.) package boneless turkey breast tenderloins
- 2 tbsp. olive oil

Directions:
1. In a small bowl, mix together the thyme, garlic powder, salt and black pepper.
2. Rub the turkey tenderloins with thyme mixture evenly.
3. Select "Sauté/Sear" setting of Ninja Foodi and place the oil into the pot.
4. Press "Start/Stop" to begin and heat for about 2-3 minutes.
5. Add the turkey tenderloins and cook, uncovered for about 10 minutes or until golden brown.
6. Press "Start/Stop" to stop cooking and transfer the turkey breast onto a plate.
7. Arrange a roasting rack into the pot. Place the turkey tenderloins over the rack.
8. Now, close the Ninja Foodi with the crisping lid and select "Bake/Roast".
9. Set the temperature to 350 degrees F for 10 minutes and press "Start/Stop" to begin.

10. Open the lid and transfer the turkey onto a cutting board for about 5 minutes before slicing. Cut into desired sized slices and serve.
- **Nutrition Info:** Calories: 162; Carbohydrates: 0.5g; Protein: 28.2g; Fat: 6.2g; Sugar: 0.1g; Sodium: 93mg; Fiber: 0.1g

68. French Style Duck Breast

Servings: 2
Cooking Time: 20 Minutes
Ingredients:
- 1 (10½-oz.) duck breast
- 1 tbsp. wholegrain mustard
- 1 tsp. honey
- 1 tsp. balsamic vinegar
- Salt and freshly ground black pepper, to taste

Directions:
1. Arrange the "Cook & Crisp Basket" in the pot of Ninja Foodi. Close the Ninja Foodi with crisping lid and select "Air Crisp". Press "Start/Stop" to begin and set the temperature to 365 degrees F. Set the time for 5 minutes to preheat.
2. Now, place the duck breast, skin side up into "Cook & Crisp Basket".
3. Close the Ninja Foodi with crisping lid and select "Air Crisp". Set the temperature to 365 degrees F for 15 minutes. Press "Start/Stop" to begin.
4. Meanwhile in a bowl, mix together remaining ingredients. Open the lid and coat the duck breast with the honey mixture generously.
5. Close the Ninja Foodi with crisping lid and set the temperature to 355 degrees F for 5 minutes. Press "Start/Stop" to begin.
6. Open the lid and serve hot.
- **Nutrition Info:** Calories: 229; Carbohydrates: 4.9g; Protein: 34.2g; Fat: 7.6g; Sugar: 3.3g; Sodium: 78mg; Fiber: 1.8g

69. Tender Chops In Sweet 'n Sour Sauce

Servings: 2
Cooking Time: 35 Minutes
Ingredients:
- 1/2 tablespoon olive oil

- 1-pound pork chops, pounded
- 1 onion, chopped
- 3 cloves of garlic minced
- 1/3 cup pineapple chunks
- 1 green bell pepper, chopped
- 1/3 cup water
- 2 tbsp ketchup
- 2 tbsp white vinegar
- 1 ½ teaspoons white sugar
- 1/2 tablespoon soy sauce
- 1 tablespoon tomato paste
- 1 teaspoon worcestershire sauce
- 1 tablespoon cornstarch + 1 1/2 tablespoons water

Directions:

1. Press the sauté button in the Ninja Foodi and heat the oil. Sear the pork chops on both sides for 5 minutes and add the onions and garlic until fragrant.
2. Stir in the rest of the ingredients except for the cornstarch and water.
3. Install pressure lid. Close Ninja Foodi, press the pressure button, choose high settings, and set time to 30 minutes.
4. Once done cooking, do a quick release.
5. Press the sauté button and stir in the cornstarch. Allow to simmer for a minute to thicken the sauce.
6. Serve and enjoy.
- **Nutrition Info:** Calories: 405; carbohydrates:35 g; protein: 46g; fat: 9g

70. Almonds Coated Lamb

Servings: 6
Cooking Time: 35 Minutes
Ingredients:

- 1¾ lb. rack of lamb
- Salt and freshly ground black pepper, to taste
- 1 egg
- 1 tbsp. breadcrumbs
- 3-oz. almonds, chopped finely

Directions:

1. Season the rack of lamb with salt and black pepper evenly and then, drizzle with cooking spray. In a shallow dish, beat the egg.

2. In another shallow dish mix together breadcrumbs and almonds.
3. Dip the rack of lamb in egg and then coat with the almond mixture.
4. Arrange the "Cook & Crisp Basket" in the pot of Ninja Foodi. Close the Ninja Foodi with crisping lid and select "Air Crisp". Press "Start/Stop" to begin and set the temperature to 220 degrees F. Set the time for 5 minutes to preheat.
5. Now, place the rack of lamb into "Cook & Crisp Basket". Close the Ninja Foodi with crisping lid and select "Air Crisp". Set the temperature to 220 degrees F for 30 minutes.
6. Press "Start/Stop" to begin. Now, set the temperature to 390 degrees F for 5 minutes. Open the lid and serve.
- **Nutrition Info:** Calories: 319; Carbohydrates: 3.9g; Protein: 31g; Fat: 19.6g; Sugar: 0.7g; Sodium: 139mg; Fiber: 1.8g

71. Spice Crusted Chicken Breasts

Servings: 4
Cooking Time: 35 Minutes
Ingredients:

- 1½ tbsp. smoked paprika
- 1 tsp. ground cumin
- Salt and freshly ground black pepper, to taste
- 2 (12-oz.) bone-in, skin-on chicken breasts
- 1 tbsp. olive oil

Directions:

1. In a small bowl, mix together paprika, cumin, salt and black pepper.
2. Coat the chicken breasts with oil evenly and then season with the spice mixture generously. Arrange the "Cook & Crisp Basket" in the pot of Ninja Foodi.
3. Close the Ninja Foodi with crisping lid and select "Air Crisp".
4. Press "Start/Stop" to begin and set the temperature to 375 degrees F.
5. Set the time for 5 minutes to preheat.
6. Now, place the chicken breasts into the "Cook & Crisp Basket".

7. Close the Ninja Foodi with crisping lid and select "Air Crisp".
8. Set the temperature to 375 degrees F for 35 minutes.
9. Press "Start/Stop" to begin。 Open the lid and transfer the chicken breasts onto a cutting board for about 5 minutes.
10. Cut each breast in 2 equal sized pieces and serve.

- **Nutrition Info:** Calories: 363; Carbohydrates: 1.7g; Protein: 49.7g; Fat: 16.6g; Sugar: 0.3g; Sodium: 187mg; Fiber: 1g

72. Short Ribs And Veggies

Servings: 4
Cooking Time: 1 Hour
Ingredients:

- 3 pounds bone in beef short ribs
- 2 tsp salt
- 1 tsp ground black pepper
- 1 cup chopped onion
- ¼ cup Marsala wine
- ½ cup beef broth
- 2 Tbsp stevia
- 4 cloves garlic, chopped
- 1 tbsp chopped thyme
- 2 parsnips, chopped
- 1 cup pearl onions
- 1 cup chopped beets

Directions:

1. Season ribs with the salt and pepper and then add to the Ninja Foodi pot with 1 Tbsp of oil. Select the sear function and let the ribs sear for 5 minutes, flip and sear for another 5 minutes.
2. Add the onion, wine, broth, stevia, garlic and thyme and place the pressure cooker lid on the Foodi. Set the pressure to high and the timer to 40 minutes. Once the timer is complete, quickly release the steam and open the lid.
3. Place the reversible rack over the top of the ribs in the pot. Place the veggies on the rack and drizzle with some extra oil.
4. Close the crisper lid and set the temperature to 350 for 15 minutes.

5. Remove the veggies and ribs and set aside. Press the sauté function and let the sauce in the pot cook for two more minutes before serving with the ribs and veggies.

- **Nutrition Info:** Calories: 506g, Carbohydrates: 14g, Protein: 47g, Fat: 27g, Sugar: 10g, Sodium: 1647 mg

73. Pulled Pork With Apple-bacon-bbq Sauce

Servings: 2
Cooking Time: 25 Minutes
Ingredients:

- 1 slice of bacon, chopped
- ½ cup onion, chopped
- 1 medium apple, chopped
- ½ cup ketchup
- 1 tablespoon sear button sugar
- 2 tbsp Worcestershire sauce
- 1 tablespoon apple cider vinegar
- 1/2 teaspoon salt
- 1-pound pork tenderloin

Directions:

1. Press the sauté button on the Ninja Foodi and add the chopped bacon. Cook until the bacon has rendered its fat. Set aside.
2. Sauté the onions and apples for a minute. Add the ketchup, sear button sugar, Worcestershire sauce, and apple cider vinegar. Season with salt.
3. Add the pork tenderloin.
4. Install pressure lid.
5. Close the lid and press the manual button. Cook on high for 25 minutes.
6. Do a complete natural pressure release.
7. Remove the pork from the pot and shred using a fork.
8. Garnish with crispy bacon.

- **Nutrition Info:** Calories: 246; carbohydrates: 19.0g; protein: 25.7g; fat: 7.4g

74. Beef Roast

Servings: 6
Cooking Time: 25 Minutes
Ingredients:

- 2 pound chuck roast
- 1 Tbsp olive oil

- 1 tsp salt
- 1 tsp ground black pepper
- 1 tsp onion powder
- 1 tsp garlic powder
- 4 cups beef stock

Directions:
1. Place the roast in the Ninja Foodi pot and season with the salt and pepper. Add the oil and then use the saute function to sear each side of the roast for 3 minutes to brown.
2. Add the beef broth, onion powder and garlic powder.
3. Close the pressure cooker lid and set the timer for high pressure, 40 minutes.
4. Once the timer has gone off, naturally release the pressure from the pot.
5. Open the lid and serve while hot.
- **Nutrition Info:** Calories: 308g, Carbohydrates: 2g, Protein: 24g, Fat: 22g, Sugar: 2g, Sodium: 1142mg

75. Everyday Chicken Breast

Servings: 4 Servings
Cooking Time: 8 Minutes
Ingredients:
- 4 boneless skinless chicken breasts
- ½ cup water

Directions:
1. Place the chicken breast in the Ninja Foodi pot and add the water.
2. Close the pressure seal lid and set the steamer valve to seal.
3. Cook on high pressure for 8 minutes then do a quick pressure release. Serve the chicken while hot.
- **Nutrition Info:** Calories: 249g, Carbohydrates: 0g, Protein: 52g, Fat: 2g, Sugar: 0g, Sodium: 149mg

76. Mild Flavored Rabbit

Servings: 6
Cooking Time: 6 Hours
Ingredients:
- 1 (4-lb.) rabbit, cut into pieces
- 12-14 whole red baby potatoes
- 8 -10 C. chicken broth
- 3 tbsp. mixed fresh herbs (thyme, basil and parsley), chopped

- Salt and freshly ground black pepper, to taste

Directions:
1. Grease the pot of Ninja Foodi generously.
2. In the prepared pot, place all the ingredients and stir to combine.
3. Close the crisping lid and select "Slow Cooker".
4. Set on "High" for about 5-6 hours.
5. Press "Start/Stop" to begin.
6. Open the lid and serve.
- **Nutrition Info:** Calories: 851; Carbohydrates: 54.1g; Protein: 100g; Fat: 26.3g; Sugar: 7g; Sodium: 800mg; Fiber: 6.5g

77. Whole Roasted Chicken

Servings: 6 Servings
Cooking Time: 40 Minutes
Ingredients:
- Whole 5 pounds Chicken
- 2 Tbsp salt
- ¼ cup lemon juice
- ¼ cup water
- 1 Tbsp stevia powder
- 1 tsp salt
- ½ tsp ground black pepper
- 1 Tbsp dried thyme
- 4 garlic cloves, minced
- 1 Tbsp olive oil

Directions:
1. Add the salt, lemon juice, water, stevia, black pepper, thyme and garlic to the Ninja Foodi Pot.
2. Place the chicken inside the pot as well and brush with the seasoning mix.
3. Move the chicken to the air crisper basket and place back into the pot.
4. Put the pressure cooker lid on the Foodi and seal. Set the pressure cooker function to high for 15 minutes. Once the cooking cycle is complete, do a quick pressure release and open the top.
5. Coat the chicken with the olive oil and put the crisper lid on and sue the air crisper function set to 400 degrees for 15 minutes.
6. Check the chicken after 15 minutes and make sure the internal temperature is 165.

7. Slice and serve while hot.
- **Nutrition Info:** Calories: 235 g, Carbohydrates: 4g, Protein: 18g, Fat: 17g, Sugar: 2g, Sodium: 592 mg

78. Mediterranean Turkey Cutlets

Servings: 4
Cooking Time: 25 Minutes
Ingredients:
- 1 tsp. Greek seasoning
- 1 lb. turkey cutlets
- 2 tbsps. olive oil
- 1 tsp. turmeric powder
- ½ c. almond flour

Directions:
1. Combine Greek seasoning, turmeric powder and almond flour in a bowl.
2. Dredge turkey cutlets in it and set aside for about 30 minutes.
3. Press "Sauté" on Ninja Foodi and add oil and turkey cutlets.
4. Sauté for about 2 minutes and add turkey cutlets.
5. Press "Pressure" and set to "Lo:Md" for about 20 minutes.
6. Dish out in a serving platter.
- **Nutrition Info:** 340 calories, 19.4g fat, 3.7g carbs, 36.3g protein

79. Bbq Turkey Legs

Servings: 6
Cooking Time: 8 Hours
Ingredients:
- 6 turkey legs
- Salt and freshly ground black pepper, to taste
- 1 C. BBQ sauce
- 2 tbsp. prepared mustard
- 1/3 C. water

Directions:
1. Season each turkey leg with salt and black pepper generously.
2. In a bowl, add remaining ingredients and mix until well combined.
3. Grease the pot of Ninja Foodi generously.
4. In the prepared pot, place the turkey legs and top with sauce evenly.

5. Close the crisping lid and select "Slow Cooker".
6. Set on "Low" for about 7-8 hours.
7. Press "Start/Stop" to begin. Open the lid and serve.
- **Nutrition Info:** Calories: 421; Carbohydrates: 15.4g; Protein: 67.2g; Fat: 8.1g; Sugar: 10.9g; Sodium: 759mg; Fiber: 0.4g

80. Creamy Tomato Chicken

Servings: 6
Cooking Time: 6 Hours
Ingredients:
- ¾ C. chicken broth
- 1 C. sour cream
- 1½ C. fresh tomatoes, chopped finely
- Salt and freshly ground black pepper, to taste
- 6 (6-oz.) boneless, skinless chicken breasts

Directions:
1. In the pot of Ninja Foodi, add all the ingredients and stir to combine.
2. Close the crisping lid and select "Slow Cooker".
3. Set on "Low" for about 6 hours.
4. Press "Start/Stop" to begin.
5. Open the lid and serve hot.
- **Nutrition Info:** Calories: 418; Carbohydrates: 3.5g; Protein: 51.4g; Fat: 20.9g; Sugar: 1.3g; Sodium: 291mg; Fiber: 0.5g

81. Texas Steak

Servings: 6
Cooking Time: 16 Minutes
Ingredients:
- 1 (2-lb.) rib eye steak
- 2 tbsp. steak rub
- 1 tbsp. olive oil
- 2 C. beef broth

Directions:
1. Season the steak with steak rub evenly and set aside for about 10 minutes.
2. Select "Sauté/Sear" setting of Ninja Foodi and place the oil into the pot.
3. Press "Start/Stop" to begin and heat for about 2-3 minutes.

4. Add the steak and cook, uncovered for about 3 minutes per side.
5. Press "Start/Stop" to stop the cooking and stir in the broth.
6. Cover the Ninja Foodi with the pressure lid and place the pressure valve to "Seal" position.
7. Select "Pressure" and set to "High" for about 10 minutes.
8. Press "Start/Stop" to begin. Switch the valve to "Vent" and do a "Quick" release.
9. Once all the pressure is released, open the lid.
10. Serve hot.
- **Nutrition Info:** Calories: 455; Carbohydrates: 1.3g; Protein: 28.4g; Fat: 36.2g; Sugar: 0.2g; Sodium: 561mg; Fiber: 0g

82. Creamy Chicken Breasts

Servings: 4
Cooking Time: 25 Minutes
Ingredients:
- 1 small onion
- 2 tbsps. butter
- 1 lb. chicken breasts
- ½ c. sour cream
- Salt

Directions:
1. Apply salt to the chicken breasts generously and keep aside.
2. Heat butter in a skillet on medium-low heat and add onions.
3. Sauté for 3 minutes and add chicken breasts.
4. Cover the lid and cook for about 10 minutes.
5. Stir in the sour cream and cook for about 4 minutes.
6. Stir gently and dish out to serve.
- **Nutrition Info:** 447 calories, 26.9g fat, 3.8g carbs, 45.3g protein

83. Mexican Style Pork Chops

Servings: 4
Cooking Time: 8 Minutes
Ingredients:
- 2 pounds pork chops
- ½ cup water
- 1 cup chopped tomatoes
- ½ cup chopped onion
- 1 jalapeno, seeds removed, minced
- 1 tbsp lime juice
- ½ tsp salt
- ¼ tsp ground black pepper

Directions:
1. Place the pork chop in the Ninja Foodi pot and add all the ingredients to the bowl.
2. Close the pressure seal lid and set the steamer valve to seal.
3. Cook on high pressure for 8 minutes then do a quick pressure release. Serve the pork while hot.
- **Nutrition Info:** Calories: 155g, Carbohydrates: 7g, Protein: 24g, Fat: 5g, Sugar: 5g, Sodium: 793 mg

84. The Shiny Chicken Stock

Servings: 4
Cooking Time: 2 Hours 10 Mins
Ingredients:
- 2 lbs. meaty chicken bones
- ¼ tsp. salt
- 3½ c. water

Directions:
1. Place chicken parts in Foodi and season with salt
2. Add water, place the pressure cooker lid and seal the valve, cook on HIGH pressure for 90 minutes
3. Release the pressure naturally over 10 minutes
4. Line a cheesecloth on a colander and place it over a large bowl, pour chicken parts and stock into the colander and strain out the chicken and bones
5. Let the stock cool and let it peel off any layer of fat that might accumulate on the surface
6. Use as needed!
- **Nutrition Info:** 51 calories, 3g fat, 2g carbs. 6g protein

85. One-pot Thai Red Curry

Servings: 2
Cooking Time: 20 Minutes
Ingredients:
- 1 1/2 tablespoon Thai red curry paste

- 1/2 can coconut milk
- 3/4-pound chicken breasts, sliced into chunks
- ¼ cup chicken broth
- 1 tablespoon fish sauce
- 1 teaspoon sear button sugar
- 1/2 tablespoon lime juice
- 1/2 cup red and green bell pepper
- 1/2 cup carrots, peeled and sliced
- ½ cup cubed onion
- 2 lime leaves
- 6 thai basil leaves

Directions:
1. Place all ingredients in the Ninja Foodi and give a good stir.
2. Install pressure lid. Close Ninja Foodi, press the manual button, choose high settings, and set time to 20 minutes.
3. Once done cooking, do a quick release.
4. Serve and enjoy.
- **Nutrition Info:** Calories: 528; carbohydrates: 15.9g; protein: 53.4g; fat: 27.8g

86. Christmas Dinner Platter

Servings: 6
Cooking Time: 8 Hours
Ingredients:
- 1 (3¼ lb.) bone-in leg of lamb
- 4-5 medium Desiree potatoes, chopped into chunks
- 1 head garlic, peeled
- Salt and freshly ground black pepper, to taste
- 1 C. wine

Directions:
1. Grease the pot of Ninja Foodi generously. Press "Start/Stop" to begin and heat for about 2-3 minutes. Add the lamb and cook, uncovered for about 10 minutes or until browned completely.
2. Press "Start/Stop" to stop the cooking and transfer the lamb onto a plate.
3. In the bottom of pot, place the potatoes and about half of the garlic cloves.
4. Place the lamb on top of the potatoes and rub with remaining garlic cloves.

5. Sprinkle with salt and black pepper and pour wine on top.
6. Close the crisping lid and select "Slow Cooker". Set on "Low" for about 6-8 hours.
7. Press "Start/Stop" to begin. Open the lid and transfer the leg of lamb onto a cutting board. Cut into desired sized pieces and serve alongside the potatoes.
- **Nutrition Info:** Calories: 946; Carbohydrates: 24.7g; Protein: 74.9g; Fat: 55.1g; Sugar: 2g; Sodium: 270mg; Fiber: 3.5g

87. Pot Roast Recipe With An Asian Twist

Servings: 2
Cooking Time: 50 Minutes
Ingredients:
- 1-pound beef pot roast
- 1/2 tablespoon Chinese five-spice powder
- ¼ cup soy sauce
- ¼ cup black bean sauce
- 2 pieces star anise
- 2 bay leaves
- 1 cup water
- 1 onion, diced
- 3 cloves of garlic, minced
- Sesame seeds for garnish

Directions:
1. Place all ingredients in the Ninja Foodi except for the sesame seeds.
2. Install pressure lid.
3. Close Ninja Foodi, press pressure button, choose high settings, and set time to 20 minutes.
4. Once done cooking, do a quick release.
5. Garnish with sesame seeds.
6. Serve and enjoy.
- **Nutrition Info:** Calories: 354; carbohydrates: 6.5; protein: 51.9g; fat: 13.3g

88. Chicken Soup

Servings: 4 Servings
Cooking Time: 8 Minutes
Ingredients:
- 1 pound chicken breast
- 4 cups chicken broth
- 2 cloves of garlic, chopped

- 1 carrot, chopped
- 2 celery stalks, chopped
- ½ white onion, chopped
- ¼ tsp salt
- 1/8 tsp ground black pepper
- ¼ cup shredded cheddar cheese

Directions:
1. Add all the ingredients to the pot and place the pressure cooker lid on the Ninja Foodi.
2. Cook on high pressure for 10 minutes. Do a quick steam release and remove the lid.
3. Shred the chicken using two forks.
4. Serve while hot or freeze to use at a later date.
- **Nutrition Info:** Calories: 217g, Carbohydrates: 2g, Protein: 33g, Fat: 4g, Sugar: 2g, Sodium: 755 mg

89. Thai Egg Rolls

Servings: 4
Cooking Time: 8 Minutes
Ingredients:
- 2 C. cooked beef, shredded
- ¼ C. Thai peanut sauce
- 1 medium carrot, peeled and julienned
- 1 red bell pepper, seeded and julienned
- 4 egg roll wrappers

Directions:
1. In a bowl, add the beef and peanut sauce and toss to coat well.
2. In another bowl, mix together the carrot and bell pepper.
3. With a damp cloth, cover the wrappers to avoid the drying.
4. Arrange 1 wrapper onto a clean, smooth surface.
5. Place about ¼ of the carrot mixture onto the bottom third of 1 wrapper, followed by ½ C. of the beef mixture. With wet fingers, moisten the outside edges of wrapper. Fold the sides of the wrapper over the filling, then roll up from the bottom.
6. Pinch the center to create a round, sausage-like roll.
7. Repeat with the remaining wrappers and filling.
8. Spray each egg roll with cooking spray evenly.
9. Arrange the "Cook & Crisp Basket" in the pot of Ninja Foodi.
10. Close the Ninja Foodi with crisping lid and select "Air Crisp".
11. Press "Start/Stop" to begin and set the temperature to 390 degrees F.
12. Set the time for 5 minutes to preheat.
13. Now, place the rolls into "Cook & Crisp Basket".
14. Close the Ninja Foodi with crisping lid and select "Air Crisp".
15. Set the temperature to 390 degrees F for 8 minutes.
16. Press "Start/Stop" to begin.
17. Open the lid and cut each roll in 2 equal sized portions before serving.
- **Nutrition Info:** Calories: 461; Carbohydrates: 42.3g; Protein: 42.8g; Fat: 12.9g; Sugar: 10.8g; Sodium: 741mg; Fiber: 2.9g

90. Garlic Creamy Beef Steak

Servings: 6
Cooking Time: 1 Hour 30 Mins
Ingredients:
- ½ c. butter
- 4 minced garlic cloves
- 2 lbs. beef top sirloin steaks
- Salt and black pepper
- 1½ c. cream

Directions:
1. Rub the beef sirloin steaks with garlic, salt and black pepper.
2. Marinate the beef with butter and cream and set aside.
3. Place grill in the Ninja Foodi and transfer the steaks on it.
4. Press "Broil" and set the timer for about 30 minutes at 365 degrees F, flipping once in the middle way.
5. Dish out and serve hot.
- **Nutrition Info:** 353 calories, 24.1g fat, 3.9g carbs, 31.8g protein

91. St. Patty's Corned Beef Recipe

Servings: 2
Cooking Time: 60 Minutes
Ingredients:

- 2 cloves of garlic, chopped
- 1/2 onion, quartered
- 1 1/4 pounds corned beef brisket, cut in large slices
- 3-oz. Beer
- 1 cup water
- 2 small carrots, roughly chopped
- 1 small potato, chopped
- 1/2 head cabbage, cut into four pieces

Directions:

1. In the Ninja Foodi, place the garlic, onion, corned beef brisket, beer, and water. Season with salt and pepper to taste.
2. Install pressure lid. Close Ninja Foodi, press the pressure button, choose high settings, and set time to 50 minutes.
3. Once done cooking, do a quick release. Open the lid and take out the meat. Shred the meat using fork and place it back into the Ninja Foodi.
4. Stir in the vegetables.
5. Install pressure lid. Close the lid and seal the vent and press the pressure button. Cook for another 10 minutes. Do quick release.
6. Serve and enjoy.
- **Nutrition Info:** Calories:758; carbohydrates: 45.8g; protein: 43.1g; fat: 44.7g

92. Ninja Foodi Salsa Verde Chicken

Servings: 2
Cooking Time: 20 Minutes
Ingredients:

- 1-pound boneless chicken breasts
- 1/4 teaspoon salt
- 1 cup commercial salsa verde

Directions:

1. Place all ingredients in the Ninja Foodi.
2. Install pressure lid. Close Ninja Foodi, press the manual button, choose high settings, and set time to 20 minutes.
3. Once done cooking, do a quick release.
4. Serve and enjoy.
- **Nutrition Info:** Calories: 273; carbohydrates: 2.5g; protein: 51.4g; fat: 6.3g

93. Ropa Vieja

Servings: 6
Cooking Time: 00 Minutes
Ingredients:

- 2 Pounds chuck roast
- 1 sliced onion
- 4 cloves garlic, minced
- 2 tsp oregano
- 1 tsp cumin
- 1 tsp paprika
- 2 tsp salt
- ½ tsp ground black pepper
- 1/8 tsp ground cloves
- 2 bay leaves
- 1 can diced tomatoes
- 2 red bell peppers

Directions:

1. Add all the ingredients to the Ninja Foodi except the green bell peppers.
2. Close the pressure cooker lid and seal the steamer valve. Set the timer for 90 minutes on low pressure.
3. Allow the pressure to naturally release and then open the lid and shred the beef with two forks.
4. Add the bell peppers and place the crisper lid on the pot. Cook at 350 for 5 minutes.
5. Serve hot
- **Nutrition Info:** Calories: 358g, Carbohydrates: 3g, Protein: 28g, Fat: 26 g, Sugar: 3g, Sodium: 855 mg

94. Breaded Chicken Tenders

Servings: 4
Cooking Time: 12 Minutes
Ingredients:

- 1 C. all-purpose flour
- 3 eggs, beaten
- 2 C. Italian bread crumbs
- 1 lb. uncooked chicken tenderloins
- Kosher salt, to taste

Directions:

1. Select "Bake/Roast" of Ninja Foodi and set the temperature to 360 degrees F.
2. Press "Start/Stop" to begin and preheat the Ninja Foodi for about 10 minutes.

3. In 3 different shallow bowls, place the flour, eggs and bread crumbs respectively.
4. Coat the chicken tenders with the flour, then dip into eggs and finally, coat with bread crumbs evenly coat. Set aside.
5. In the pot of Ninja Foodi, arrange the reversible rack.
6. Arrange the chicken tenders over the rack, without overlapping.
7. Close the Ninja Foodi with the crisping lid and set time for 12 minutes.
8. Press "Start/Stop" to begin.
9. Open the lid and serve hot with the sprinkling of salt.
- **Nutrition Info:** Calories: 477; Carbohydrates: 64.1g; Protein: 38.3g; Fat: 7.2g; Sugar: 4.4g; Sodium: 1200mg; Fiber: 2.8g

95. Aromatic Roasted Chicken

Servings: 7
Cooking Time: 1 Hour 29 Minutes
Ingredients:
- 1 (6-lb.) whole chicken, necks and giblets removed
- Salt and freshly ground black pepper, to taste
- 3 fresh rosemary sprigs, divided
- 1 lemon, zested and cut into quarters
- 2 large onions, sliced,
- 4 C. chicken broth

Directions:
1. Stuff the cavity of chicken with 2 rosemary sprigs and lemon quarters.
2. Season the chicken with salt and black pepper evenly. Chop the remaining rosemary sprig and set aside.
3. Select "Sauté/Sear" setting of Ninja Foodi and place the chicken into the pot.
4. Press "Start/Stop" to begin and cook, uncovered for about 5-7 minutes per side.
5. Remove chicken from the pot and arrange onto a roasting rack.
6. In the pot, place the onions and broth. Arrange the roasting rack into the pot and sprinkle the chicken with reserved chopped rosemary and lemon zest.

7. Close the Ninja Foodi with the crisping lid and select "Bake/Roast".
8. Set the temperature to 375 degrees F for 1¼ hours and press "Start/Stop" to begin. Open the lid and transfer the chicken onto a cutting board for about 10 minutes before carving.
9. Cut into desired sized pieces and serve.
- **Nutrition Info:** Calories: 628; Carbohydrates: 5.1g; Protein: 116g; Fat: 12.7g; Sugar: 2.3g; Sodium: 706mg; Fiber: 1.2g

96. Chicken Taco Filling

Servings: 8
Cooking Time: 4 Hours
Ingredients:
- ¼ C. low-sodium soy sauce
- ¼ C. blackberry jam
- ¼ C. honey
- ½ tsp. red pepper flakes, crushed
- 5 (8-oz.) boneless, skinless chicken breasts

Directions:
1. Grease the pot of Ninja Foodi generously.
2. In a bowl, add all the ingredients except the chicken breasts and mix well.
3. In the prepared pot, place the chicken breasts and top with the honey mixture.
4. Close the crisping lid and select "Slow Cooker".
5. Set on "High" for about 4 hours.
6. Press "Start/Stop" to begin.
7. Open the lid and with 2 forks, shred the meat and stir with sauce well.
8. Serve hot.
- **Nutrition Info:** Calories: 329; Carbohydrates: 15.8g; Protein: 41.6g; Fat: 10.5g; Sugar: 15.2g; Sodium: 562mg; Fiber: 0.1g

97. Zingy Chicken Wings

Servings: 4
Cooking Time: 20 Minutes
Ingredients:
- 1 tbsp. fish sauce
- 1 tbsp. fresh lemon juice
- 1 tsp. sugar

- Salt and freshly ground black pepper, to taste
- 12 chicken middle wings, cut into half

Directions:
1. In In a bowl, mix together fish sauce, lime juice, sugar, salt and black pepper.
2. Add wings ad coat with mixture generously. Refrigerate to marinate for about 1 hour.
3. In the pot of Ninja Foodi, place 1 C. of water.
4. Place the chicken wings into "Cook & Crisp Basket". Arrange the "Cook & Crisp Basket" in the pot. Cover the Ninja Foodi with the pressure lid and place the pressure valve to "Seal" position.
5. Select "Pressure" and set to "High" for about 5 minutes. Press "Start/Stop" to begin. Switch the valve to "Vent" and do a "Quick" release.
6. Once all the pressure is released, open the lid
7. Now, close the Ninja Foodi with the crisping lid and select "Air Crisp".
8. Set the temperature to 390 degrees F for 13-15 minutes. Press "Start/Stop" to begin. After 7 minutes, flip the wings.
9. Meanwhile, in a large bowl, add Buffalo sauce and salt and mix well.
10. Open the lid and transfer the wings into the bowl of Buffalo sauce.
11. Then, toss the wings well to coat with the Buffalo sauce.
12. Serve immediately.
- **Nutrition Info:** Calories: 483; Carbohydrates: 17.3g; Protein: 29.5g; Fat: 32.1g; Sugar: 1.2g; Sodium: 857mg; Fiber: 0.5g

98. Luscious Chicken Breasts

Servings: 4
Cooking Time: 20 Minutes
Ingredients:
- 2 (8-oz.) skinless, boneless chicken fillets
- Salt and freshly ground black pepper, to taste
- 4 brie cheese slices
- 1 tbsp. fresh chive, minced
- 4 cured ham slices

Directions:

1. Cut each chicken fillet in 2 equal sized pieces.
2. Carefully, make a slit in each chicken piece horizontally about ¼-inch from the edge.
3. Open each chicken piece and season with the salt and black pepper.
4. Place 1 cheese slice in the open area of each chicken piece and sprinkle with chives.
5. In the pot of Ninja Foodi, place 1 C. of water.
6. Place the rolled chicken breasts into "Cook & Crisp Basket".
7. Arrange the "Cook & Crisp Basket" in the pot.
8. Cover the Ninja Foodi with the pressure lid and place the pressure valve to "Seal" position. Select "Pressure" and set to "High" for about 5 minutes.
9. Press "Start/Stop" to begin. Switch the valve to "Vent" and do a "Quick" release.
10. Once all the pressure is released, open the lid
11. Now, close the Ninja Foodi with the crisping lid and Select "Air Crisp".
12. Set the temperature to 355 degrees F for 15 minutes. Press "Start/Stop" to begin.
13. Open the lid and transfer the rolled chicken breasts onto a cutting board.
14. Cut into desired sized slices and serve.
- **Nutrition Info:** Calories: 271; Carbohydrates: 1.2g; Protein: 35.2g; Fat: 13.4g; Sugar: 0.1g; Sodium: 602mg; Fiber: 0.4g

99. Ginger-balsamic Glazed Chicken

Servings: 2
Cooking Time: 15 Minutes
Ingredients:
- 4 chicken thighs, skinless
- 1/4 cup balsamic vinegar
- 1 1/2 tablespoons mustard
- 1 tablespoon ginger garlic paste
- 4 cloves of garlic, minced
- 1-inch fresh ginger root
- 2 tablespoons honey
- Salt and pepper to taste

Directions:
1. Place all ingredients in the Ninja Foodi. Stir to combine everything.

2. Install pressure lid. Close Ninja Foodi, press the manual button, choose high settings, and set time to 15 minutes.
3. Once done cooking, do a quick release. Remove pressure lid.
4. Mix and turnover chicken.
5. Cover, press roast, and roast for 5 minutes.
6. Serve and enjoy.
- **Nutrition Info:** Calories: 476; carbohydrates:12.5g; protein: 32.4g; fat: 32.9g

100.Sausage 'n Spinach Sweet Potato Hash

Servings: 2
Cooking Time: 40 Minutes
Ingredients:
- 2 medium sweet potatoes, peeled and cut into 1-inch pieces
- 1 tablespoon olive oil, divided
- 1/2 teaspoon kosher salt
- 6-ounces Italian sausage
- 1 small onion, finely chopped
- 2 cloves garlic, minced or put through a garlic press
- 1/2 teaspoon ground sage
- 1/4 teaspoon freshly ground black pepper
- 5-ounces baby spinach
- 2 large eggs

Directions:
1. Preheat Ninja Foodi to 425 ºF for 5 minutes.
2. On the Ninja Foodi pot, add sweet potatoes and drizzle with salt and 2 teaspoons olive oil. Roast for 20 minutes or until fork tender. Midway through roasting time, stir potatoes. Once done roasting turn oven off and set sweet potatoes aside.
3. Press sauté button on Ninja Foodi and heat remaining oil. Sauté sausage and crumble to pieces. Cook for 10 minutes.
4. Stir in pepper, sage, garlic, and onions. Sauté for three minutes.
5. Stir in spinach and sweet potatoes and mix well.
6. Break eggs on top of the mixture.
7. Close Ninja Foodi, press bake button, bake at 350 ºF for 5 minutes.
8. Serve and enjoy.

- **Nutrition Info:** Calories: 510; carbohydrates: 29.2g; protein: 26.6g; fat: 31.9g

101.Beef Jerky

Servings: 6
Cooking Time: 10 Minutes
Ingredients:
- ½ pound beef, sliced into 1/8" Thick strips
- ½ cup soy sauce
- 2 Tbsp Worcestershire sauce
- 2 tsp ground black pepper
- 1 tsp onion powder
- ½ tsp garlic powder
- 1 tsp kosher salt

Directions:
1. Place all the ingredients in a large Ziploc bag and seal shut. Shake to mix. Leave in the fridge overnight.
2. Lay the strips on the dehydrator trays, being careful not to overlap them.
3. Place the cook and crisp lid on and set the temperature for 135 degrees for 7 hours. Once done, store in an airtight container.

- **Nutrition Info:** Calories: 62g, Carbohydrates: 2g, Protein: 9g, Fat: 1g, Sugar: 1g, Sodium: 1482 mg

102.Beef Stew

Servings: 4
Cooking Time: 10 Minutes
Ingredients:
- 1 pound Beef Roast
- 4 cups beef broth
- 3 cloves of garlic, chopped
- 1 carrot, chopped
- 2 celery stalks, chopped
- 2 tomatoes, chopped
- ½ white onion, chopped
- ¼ tsp salt
- 1/8 tsp ground black pepper

Directions:
1. Add all the ingredients to the pot and place the pressure cooker lid on the Ninja Foodi.
2. Cook on high pressure for 10 minutes. Do a quick steam release and remove the lid.
3. Shred the chicken using two forks.

4. Serve while hot or freeze to use at a later date.
- **Nutrition Info:** Calories: 211g, Carbohydrates: 2g, Protein: 10g, Fat: 7g, Sugar: 2g, Sodium: 147 mg

103.Potatoes, Beefy-cheesy Way

Servings: 2
Cooking Time: 25 Minutes
Ingredients:
- ½ pounds ground beef
- 2 large potatoes, peeled and chopped
- 3/4 cup cheddar cheese, shredded
- 1/4 cup chicken broth
- 1/2 tablespoon Italian seasoning mix
- Salt and pepper to taste

Directions:
1. Press the sauté button on the Ninja Foodi and stir in the beef. Sear button the meat until some of the oil has rendered.
2. Add the rest of the ingredients.
3. Install pressure lid.
4. Close Ninja Foodi, press the pressure button, choose high settings, and set time to 20 minutes.
5. Once done cooking, do a quick release.
6. Serve and enjoy.
- **Nutrition Info:** Calories: 801; carbohydrates: 66.8g; protein: 53.4g; fat: 35.6g

104.Cauliflower Corned Beef Hash

Servings: 6
Cooking Time: 30 Minutes
Ingredients:
- 6 eggs
- 4 cups riced cauliflower
- 1 pound corned beef, diced
- ¼ cup milk
- 1 onion, chopped
- 3 Tbsp butter
- 2 cups chopped, cooked ham
- ½ cup shredded cheese

Directions:
1. Press the saute button on your Ninja Foodi and add the butter and the onions. Cook, stirring occasionally until the onions are soft, about 5 minutes.

2. Add the riced cauliflower to the pot and stir. Turn on the air crisper for 15 minutes, turning the cauliflower halfway through.
3. In a small bowl, mix the eggs and milk together then pour over the browned cauliflower.
4. Sprinkle the corned beef over the top of the egg mix.
5. Press the air crisp button again and set the timer for 10 minutes.
6. Sprinkle the cheddar cheese on top and close the lid of the Ninja Foodi for one minute to just melt the cheese. Serve while hot
- **Nutrition Info:** Calories: 322g, Carbohydrates: 3g , Protein: 20g, Fat: 26 g, Sugar: 1, Sodium: 1008 mg

105.Spicy Chicken Jerky

Servings: 6 Servings
Cooking Time: 10 Minutes
Ingredients:
- ½ pound Chicken breast, sliced into 1/8" Thick strips
- ½ cup soy sauce
- 2 Tbsp Worcestershire sauce
- 2 tsp ground black pepper
- 1 tsp liquid smoke
- 1 tsp onion powder
- 1 tsp cayenne pepper
- ½ tsp garlic powder
- 1 tsp kosher salt

Directions:
1. Place all the ingredients in a large Ziploc bag and seal shut. Shake to mix. Leave in the fridge overnight.
2. Lay the strips on the dehydrator trays, being careful not to overlap them.
3. Place the cook and crisp lid on and set the temperature for 135 degrees for 7 hours. Once done, store in an airtight containers.
- **Nutrition Info:** Calories: 42g, Carbohydrates: 2g, Protein: 4g, Fat: 1g, Sugar: 1g, Sodium: 1493 mg

106.Thanksgiving Dinner Turkey

Servings: 8
Cooking Time: 1 Hour 23 Minutes

Ingredients:

- ¼ C. butter
- 5-6 carrots, peeled and cut into chunks
- 1 (6-lb.) boneless turkey breast
- Salt and freshly ground black pepper, to taste
- 1-2 C. chicken broth

Directions:

1. Select "Sauté/Sear" setting of Ninja Foodi and place the butter into the pot.
2. Press "Start/Stop" to begin and heat for about 2-3 minutes.
3. Add the carrots and cook, uncovered for about 4-5 minutes.
4. Add turkey breast and cook for about 10-15 minutes or until golden brown from both sides.
5. Press "Start/Stop" to stop cooking and stir in salt, black pepper and broth.
6. Close the Ninja Foodi with the crisping lid and select "Bake/Roast".
7. Set the temperature to 375 degrees F for 1 hour and press "Start/Stop" to begin.
8. Open the lid and transfer the turkey onto a cutting board for about 5 minutes before slicing.
9. Cut into desired sized slices and serve alongside carrots.
- **Nutrition Info:** Calories: 402; Carbohydrates: 3.9g; Protein: 8.3g; Fat: 7.4g; Sugar: 2g; Sodium: 347mg; Fiber: 0.9g

107.Not Your Ordinary Beef Pot Pie

Servings: 2
Cooking Time: 25 Minutes
Ingredients:

- 1 1/2 tablespoons butter
- 1/2 cup diced onion
- 1/2 cup diced celery
- 2 cloves of garlic, minced
- 6-oz beef
- 1 teaspoon dried thyme
- 3/4 cup potatoes, diced
- 1/3 cup carrots, diced
- 1/3 cup frozen peas
- 3/4 cups beef broth
- 2 tbsp milk

- 1 tablespoon cornstarch + 1 1/2 tablespoons water
- 1/2 box puff pastry
- 1 egg white

Directions:

1. Press the sauté button on the Ninja Foodi and heat the butter. Sauté the onion, celery and garlic until fragrant. Add the beef and sear button for 5 minutes.
2. Stir in the thyme, potatoes, carrots, frozen peas, beef broth and milk.
3. Install pressure lid. Close Ninja Foodi, press pressure button, choose high settings, and set time to 10 minutes.
4. Once done cooking, do a quick release.
5. Ladle into two ramekins and cover the top of the ramekins with puff pastry. Brush the top with egg whites.
6. Place in Ninja Foodi, bake at 350 ºF for 10 minutes or until tops are lightly browned.
7. Serve and enjoy.
- **Nutrition Info:** Calories: 328; carbohydrates: 26.6g; protein: 20.8g; fat: 15.3g

108.Glazed Turkey Breast

Servings: 7
Cooking Time:1 Hour 54 Minutes
Ingredients:

- 1 (5-lb.) boneless turkey breast
- Salt and freshly ground black pepper, to taste
- ¼ C. maple syrup
- 2 tbsp. Dijon mustard
- 1 tbsp. butter, softened

Directions:

1. Season the turkey breast with salt and black pepper generously and spray with cooking spray.
2. Arrange the "Cook & Crisp Basket" in the pot of Ninja Foodi.
3. Close the Ninja Foodi with crisping lid and select "Air Crisp".
4. Press "Start/Stop" to begin and set the temperature to 350 degrees F.
5. Set the time for 5 minutes to preheat.
6. Now, place the turkey breast into "Cook & Crisp Basket".

7. Close the Ninja Foodi with the crisping lid and Select "Air Crisp".
8. Set the temperature to 350 degrees F for 50 minutes.
9. Press "Start/Stop" to begin. Flip twice, first after 25 minutes and then after 37 minutes.
10. Meanwhile, for glaze: in a bowl, mix together the maple syrup, mustard and butter.
11. Press "Start/Stop" to stop cooking and coat the turkey with the glaze evenly.
12. Close the Ninja Foodi with the crisping lid and Select "Air Crisp".
13. Set the temperature to 350 degrees F for 5 minutes.
14. Press "Start/Stop" to begin.
15. Open the lid and transfer the turkey onto a cutting board for about 5 minutes before slicing.
16. Cut into desired sized slices and serve.
- **Nutrition Info:** Calories: 362; Carbohydrates: 7.8g; Protein: 8.5g; Fat: 3.3g; Sugar: 6.7g; Sodium: 244mg; Fiber: 0.2g

109.Out Of World Deer

Servings: 10
Cooking Time: 2½ Hours
Ingredients:
- 3-4 lb. deer, thawed
- Salt and freshly ground black pepper, to taste
- 1 (12-oz.) can beer
- ¼ C. Worcestershire sauce
- 1 tbsp. honey

Directions:
1. Grease the pot of Ninja Foodi generously.
2. Select "Sauté/Sear" setting of Ninja Foodi and place the deer meat.
3. Press "Start/Stop" to begin and cook, uncovered for about 15 minutes per side.
4. Press "Start/Stop" to stop the cooking and stir in the remaining ingredients.
5. Close the crisping lid and select "Slow Cooker".

6. Set on "High" for about 2 hours.
7. Press "Start/Stop" to begin.
8. Open the lid and with 2 forks, shred the meat.
9. Serve hot.
- **Nutrition Info:** Calories: 242; Carbohydrates: 4.1g; Protein: 41.3g; Fat: 4.3g; Sugar: 2.9g; Sodium: 156mg; Fiber: 0g

110.Beefy Stew Recipe From Persia

Servings: 2
Cooking Time: 20 Minutes
Ingredients:
- 1 tablespoons vegetable oil
- 1 onion, chopped
- 2 cloves of garlic, minced
- ¾-pound beef stew meat, cut into chunks
- 1/2 tablespoon ground cumin
- 1/4 teaspoon saffron threads
- ½ teaspoon turmeric
- ¼ teaspoon ground cinnamon
- ¼ teaspoon ground allspice
- Salt and pepper to taste
- 2 tbsp tomato paste
- 1/2 can split peas, rinsed and drained
- 2 cups bone broth
- 1 can crushed tomatoes
- 2 tablespoon lemon juice, freshly squeezed

Directions:
1. Press the sauté button on the Ninja Foodi. Heat the oil and sauté the onion and garlic until fragrant. Add cumin, saffron, turmeric, cinnamon, and allspice. Stir in the beef and sear button for 3 minutes. Season with salt and pepper to taste.
2. Pour in the rest of the ingredients.
3. Install pressure lid. Close Ninja Foodi, press the pressure button, choose high settings, and set time to 20 minutes.
4. Once done cooking, do a quick release.
5. Serve and enjoy.
- **Nutrition Info:** Calories: 466; carbohydrates: 36g; protein: 49g; fat: 14g

FISH AND SEAFOOD RECIPES

111.Cod Topped With Mediterranean-spiced Tomatoes

Servings: 6
Cooking Time: 10 Minutes
Ingredients:

- 2 frozen or fresh cod fillet
- 1 tablespoon butter
- 1/2 lemon, juiced
- ½ small onion, sliced thinly
- 1/4 teaspoon salt
- 1/4 teaspoon black pepper
- 1/2 teaspoon oregano
- ¼ tsp cumin
- ¼ tsp rosemary
- 4 roma tomatoes, diced
- ¼ cup water

Directions:

1. Press sauté and melt butter. Stir in lemon juice, onion, salt, black pepper, oregano cumin, rosemary, and diced tomatoes. Cook for 8 minutes.
2. Add fish and spoon sauce over it. Add water and press stop.
3. Install pressure lid and place valve to vent position.
4. Close Ninja Foodi, press steam button, and set time to 2 minutes.
5. Once done cooking, do a quick release. Serve and enjoy.
- **Nutrition Info:** Calories: 184; carbohydrates: 10.0g; protein: 20.7g; fat: 6.8g

112.Black Pepper Scallops

Servings: 4 Servings
Cooking Time: 17 Minutes
Ingredients:

- 2 pounds Sea Scallops
- 2 Tbsp Butter
- 1 tsp garlic powder
- 1 tsp ground black pepper
- ¼ cup lemon juice

Directions:

1. Place the scallops and butter in the pot and press saute. Sear both sides of the shrimp for 2 minutes.
2. Sprinkle the chili powder, garlic powder and ground black pepper on the shrimp and mix. Sprinkle the cheese over the shrimp and place the air crisp lid on top.
3. Use the roast function set to 400 to cook the shrimp for 15 more minutes. Serve hot.
- **Nutrition Info:** Calories: 236 g, Carbohydrates: 11g, Protein: 34g, Fat: 7g, Sugar: 0g, Sodium: 1181 mg

113.Spicy Flounder

Servings: 2 Servings
Cooking Time: 15 Minutes
Ingredients:

- 2 tsp salt
- 1 Tbsp paprika
- 1 tbsp chili powder
- 1 tsp ground black pepper
- 1 tsp onion powder
- 1 tsp garlic powder
- 1 tsp ground cumin
- 2 filets Flounder, about 1 pound
- 1 tbsp olive oil

Directions:

1. Mix all of the spices together in a bowl and then set aside.
2. Rub the flounder with the olive oil and then coat in the spice seasoning.
3. Place the spiced flounder in the cook and crisp basket and turn the Ninja Foodi to 375 degrees. Place the basket in the Foodi and set the timer for 15 minutes. Serve while hot straight out of the pot.
- **Nutrition Info:** Calories: 351g, Carbohydrates: 6g, Protein: 51g, Fat: 12g, Sugar: 6g, Sodium: 2658 mg

114.Cajun Spiced Salmon

Servings: 2
Cooking Time: 8 Minutes
Ingredients:

- 2 (6-oz.) salmon steaks
- 2 tbsp. Cajun seasoning

Directions:

1. Rub the salmon steaks with the Cajun seasoning evenly and set aside for about 10 minutes.
2. Arrange the "Cook & Crisp Basket" in the pot of Ninja Foodi.
3. Close the Ninja Foodi with crisping lid and select "Air Crisp".
4. Press "Start/Stop" to begin and set the temperature to 390 degrees F.
5. Set the time for 5 minutes to preheat.
6. Now, place the salmon steaks into "Cook & Crisp Basket".
7. Close the Ninja Foodi with crisping lid and select "Air Crisp".
8. Set the temperature to 390 degrees F for 4 minutes per side.
9. Press "Start/Stop" to begin.
10. Open the lid and serve.
- **Nutrition Info:** Calories: 225; Carbohydrates: 0g; Protein: 33.1g; Fat: 10.5g; Sugar: 0g; Sodium: 225mg; Fiber: 0g

115.Paprika Shrimp

Servings: 3
Cooking Time: 20 Minutes
Ingredients:
- 1 tsp. paprika, smoked
- 3 tbsps. butter
- 1 lb. tiger shrimps
- Salt

Directions:
1. In a bowl, mix all the above ingredients and marinate the shrimps in it.
2. Grease the pot of Ninja Foodi with butter and transfer the seasoned shrimps in it.
3. Press "Bake/Roast" and set the timer to 15 minutes at 355 degrees F.
4. Dish out shrimps from the Ninja Foodi and serve.
- **Nutrition Info:** 173 calories, 8.3g fat, 0.1g carbs, 23.8g protein

116.Tomato Lime Tilapia

Servings: 2 Servings
Cooking Time: 5 Minutes
Ingredients:
- 2 Tbsp butter
- 1/3 cup lime juice

- 1 tomato, diced
- 1 pound Salmon, de boned
- ½ tsp salt
- ¼ tsp ground black pepper

Directions:
1. Add the tilapia into the cook and crisp basket and place the basket inside the Ninja Foodi.
2. Sprinkle the seasoning over the top of the fish and then add the tomatoes, butter and lime juice around the filets.
3. Place the pressure cooker lid on top of the pot and close the pressure valve to the seal position. Set the pressure cooker function to high heat and set the timer for 3 minutes.
4. Once the cooking cycle is complete, release the pressure quickly by carefully opening the steamer valve. Enjoy while hot
- **Nutrition Info:** Calories: 317g, Carbohydrates: 9g, Protein: 42g, Fat: 14g, Sugar: 4g, Sodium: 1726mg

117.Hearty Tilapia Bowl

Servings: 2
Cooking Time: 18 Minutes
Ingredients:
- 3 C. chicken broth
- 1 C. stone ground grits
- 1 C. heavy cream
- Salt, to taste
- 2 (4-oz.) tilapia fillets

Directions:
1. In the pot of Ninja Foodi, place the chicken broth, grits, heavy cream and salt and stir to combine.
2. Cover the Ninja Foodi with the pressure lid and place the pressure valve to "Seal" position. Select "Pressure" and set to "High" for about 8 minutes.
3. Press "Start/Stop" to begin. Switch the valve to "Vent" and do a "Natural" release for about 10 minutes. Then do a "Quick" release.
4. Meanwhile, spray the tilapia fillets with cooking oil spray and then, season with salt evenly.
5. Once all the pressure is released, open the lid and stir the grits mixture.

6. Arrange a large piece of fil over grits mixture.
7. Arrange the tilapia fillets over foil in a single layer.
8. Now, close the Ninja Foodi with crisping lid and select "Air Crisp".
9. Set the temperature to 400 degrees F for 10 minutes.
10. Press "Start/Stop" to begin. Open the lid and serve the tilapia fillets with grits mixture.
- **Nutrition Info:** Calories: 679; Carbohydrates: 72g; Protein: 37.7g; Fat: 29.2g; Sugar: 1.1g; Sodium: 1300mg; Fiber: 6g

118.Sweet And Sour Fish

Servings: 3
Cooking Time: 16 Minutes
Ingredients:
- 2 drops liquid stevia
- ¼ c. butter
- 1 lb. fish chunks
- 1 tbsp. vinegar
- Salt and black pepper

Directions:
1. Press "Sauté" on Ninja Foodi and add butter and fish chunks.
2. Sauté for about 3 minutes and add stevia, salt and black pepper.
3. Press "Air Crisp" and cook for about 3 minutes at 360 degrees F.
4. Dish out in a serving bowl and serve immediately.
- **Nutrition Info:** 274 calories, 15.4 fat, 2.8g carbs, 33.2g protein

119.Shrimp Magic

Servings: 3
Cooking Time: 25 Minutes
Ingredients:
- 2 tbsps. butter
- ½ tsp. paprika, smoked
- 1 lb. deveined shrimps, peeled
- Lemongrass stalks
- 1 chopped red chili pepper, seeded

Directions:

1. In a bowl, combine all the ingredients except lemongrass and marinate for about 1 hour.
2. Press "Bake/Roast" and set the timer to 15 minutes at 345 degrees F.
3. Bake for about 15 minutes and dish out the fillets.
- **Nutrition Info:** 251 calories, 10.3g fat, 3g carbs, 34.6g protein

120.Stewed Mixed Seafood

Servings: 2
Cooking Time: 35 Minutes
Ingredients:
- 1 tbsp vegetable oil
- ½ 14.5-oz can fire-roasted tomatoes
- 1/2 cup diced onion
- 1/2 cup chopped carrots, or 1 cup chopped bell pepper
- 1/2 cup water
- 1/2 cup white wine or broth
- 1 bay leaf
- 1/2 tablespoon tomato paste
- 1 tablespoon minced garlic
- 1 teaspoon fennel seeds toasted and ground
- 1/2 teaspoon dried oregano
- 1 teaspoon salt
- 1 teaspoon red pepper flakes
- 2 cups mixed seafood such as fish chunks, shrimp, bay scallops, mussels and calamari rings, defrosted
- 1 tablespoon fresh lemon juice

Directions:
1. Press sauté button on Ninja Foodi and heat oil. Once hot, stir in onion and garlic. Sauté for 5 minutes. Stir in tomatoes, bay leaves, tomato paste, oregano, salt, and pepper flakes. Cook for 5 minutes. Press stop.
2. Stir in bell pepper, water, wine, and fennel seeds. Mix well.
3. Install pressure lid. Close Ninja Foodi, press pressure button, choose high settings, and set time to 15 minutes.
4. Once done cooking, do a quick release.
5. Stir in defrosted mixed seafood. Cover and let it cook for 10 minutes in residual heat.
6. Serve and enjoy with a dash of lemon juice.

- **Nutrition Info:** Calories: 202; carbohydrates: 10.0g; protein: 18.0g; fat: 10.0g

121.Creamy Herb 'n Parm Salmon

Servings: 2
Cooking Time: 10 Minutes
Ingredients:

- 2 frozen salmon filets
- 1/2 cup water
- 1 1/2 tsp minced garlic
- 1/4 cup heavy cream
- 1 cup parmesan cheese grated
- 1 tbsp chopped fresh chives
- 1 tbsp chopped fresh parsley
- 1 tbsp fresh dill
- 1 tsp fresh lemon juice
- Salt and pepper to taste

Directions:

1. Add water and trivet in pot. Place fillets on top of trivet.
2. Install pressure lid. Close Ninja Foodi, press pressure button, choose high settings, and set time to 4 minutes.
3. Once done cooking, do a quick release.
4. Transfer salmon to a serving plate. And remove trivet.
5. Press stop and then press sauté button on Ninja Foodi. Stir in heavy cream once water begins to boil. Boil for 3 minutes. Press stop and then stir in lemon juice, parmesan cheese, dill, parsley, and chives. Season with pepper and salt to taste. Pour over salmon.
6. Serve and enjoy.

- **Nutrition Info:** Calories: 423; carbohydrates: 6.4g; protein: 43.1g; fat: 25.0g

122.Jambalaya

Servings: 4 Servings
Cooking Time: 10 Minutes
Ingredients:

- 1 pound shrimp, deveined, shells removed
- 2 cups chicken broth
- 2 cloves of garlic, chopped
- 2 bell peppers, chopped
- 1 white onion, chopped
- 4 tomatoes, chopped

- 1 tsp dried basil
- 1 tsp dried oregano
- ½ tsp tsp salt
- 1/8 tsp ground black pepper
- ¼ cup shredded cheddar cheese

Directions:

1. Place the shrimp in the Ninja Foodi pot and sprinkle with the oregano, salt, basil and ground black pepper.
2. Add the broth, garlic, tomato, bell pepper and onion to the pot and close the pressure cooker lid.
3. Cook on high pressure for 10 minutes. Do a quick steam release and remove the lid.
4. Add the cream cheese and heavy cream and stir to blend.
5. Sprinkle the cheese on top of the chili and put the air crisper top on. Use the broil function to brown the cheese for 2 minutes.

- **Nutrition Info:** Calories: 150g, Carbohydrates: 2g, Protein: 36g, Fat: 0g, Sugar: 2g, Sodium: 438mg

123.Ketogenic Butter Fish

Servings: 3
Cooking Time: 40 Minutes
Ingredients:

- 1 lb. salmon fillets
- 2 tbsps. ginger-garlic paste
- 3 chopped green chilies
- Salt and black pepper
- ¾ c. butter

Directions:

1. Season the salmon fillets with ginger-garlic paste, salt and black pepper.
2. Place the salmon fillets in the pot of Ninja Foodi and top with green chilies and butter.
3. Press "Bake/Roast" and set the timer to 30 minutes at 360 degrees F.
4. Bake for about 30 minutes and dish out the fillets in a serving platter.

- **Nutrition Info:** 507 calories, 45.9g fat, 2.4g carbs, 22.8g protein

124.Pasta 'n Tuna Bake

Servings: 2
Cooking Time: 10 Minutes
Ingredients:

- 1 can cream-of-mushroom soup
- 1 1/2 cups water
- 1 1/4 cups macaroni pasta
- 1 can tuna
- 1/2 cup frozen peas
- 1/2 tsp salt
- 1 tsp pepper
- 1/2 cup shredded cheddar cheese

Directions:
1. Mix soup and water in Ninja Foodi.
2. Add remaining ingredients except for cheese. Stir.
3. Install pressure lid.
4. Close Ninja Foodi, press pressure button, choose high settings, and set time to 4 minutes.
5. Once done cooking, do a quick release.
6. Remove pressure lid.
7. Stir in cheese and roast for 5 minutes.
8. Serve and enjoy.
- **Nutrition Info:** Calories: 378; carbohydrates: 34.0g; protein: 28.0g; fat: 14.1g

125.Tilapia Filet Topped With Mango-salsa

Servings: 2
Cooking Time: 5 Minutes
Ingredients:
- 1 cup coconut milk
- 1/2 to 1 tablespoon Thai green curry paste
- 1 tablespoon fish sauce
- Zest of 1 lime and juice of 1/2 lime
- 2 teaspoons sear button sugar
- 1 teaspoon garlic, minced
- 1 tablespoon fresh ginger, minced
- 2 6-oz Tilapia filet
- 1 lime, cut in thin slices
- A sprinkle of cilantro leaves and chopped scallion
- Mango salsa ingredients:
- 1 mango, peeled, seeded, and diced (about 3/4 cup small dice)
- 1 fresno or jalapeno chiles, minced
- 1 scallion, finely chopped
- A handful of cilantro leaves, chopped
- Juice of 1 lime

Directions:
1. In a bowl, mix well coconut milk, Thai green curry paste, fish sauce, lime juice, lime zest, sear button sugar, garlic, and ginger. Add fish and marinate for at least an hour.
2. Meanwhile, make the mango salsa by combining all ingredients in a separate bowl. Keep in the fridge.
3. Cut two 11x11-inch foil. Place one fish fillet in each foil. Top each equally with lime, scallion and cilantro. Seal foil packets.
4. Add a cup of water in Ninja Foodi, place trivet, and add foil packets on trivet.
5. Install pressure lid. Close Ninja Foodi, press pressure button, choose high settings, and set time to 5 minutes.
6. Once done cooking, do a quick release. Serve and enjoy with mango salsa on top.
- **Nutrition Info:** Calories: 372; carbohydrates: 28.5g; protein: 29.3g; fat: 15.6g

126.Well-seasoned Catfish

Servings: 4
Cooking Time: 23 Minutes
Ingredients:
- 4 (4-oz.) catfish fillets
- ¼ C. Louisiana fish fry seasoning
- 1 tbsp. olive oil
- 1 tbsp. fresh parsley, chopped

Directions:
1. Rub the fish filets with seasoning generously and then, coat with oil.
2. Arrange the "Cook & Crisp Basket" in the pot of Ninja Foodi.
3. Close the Ninja Foodi with crisping lid and select "Air Crisp".
4. Press "Start/Stop" to begin and set the temperature to 400 degrees F.
5. Set the time for 5 minutes to preheat.
6. Now, place the fish fillets into "Cook & Crisp Basket".
7. Close the Ninja Foodi with crisping lid and select "Air Crisp".
8. Set the temperature to 400 degrees F for 23 minutes.
9. Press "Start/Stop" to begin.

10. After 10 minutes, flip the fish fillets and again after 20 minutes.
11. Open the lid and serve with the garnishing of parsley.
- **Nutrition Info:** Calories: 206; Carbohydrates: 4.7g; Protein: 17.7g; Fat: 12.1g; Sugar: 0g; Sodium: 201mg; Fiber: 0.7g

127.Flavorsome Salmon

Servings: 2
Cooking Time: 13 Minutes
Ingredients:
- ¼ C. soy sauce
- ¼ C. honey
- 2 tsp. rice wine vinegar
- 1 tsp. water
- 2 (4-oz.) salmon fillets

Directions:
1. In a small bowl, mix together all ingredients except salmon.
2. In a small bowl, reserve about half of the mixture. Add the salmon in remaining mixture and coat well. Refrigerate, covered to marinate for about 2 hours.
3. Arrange the "Cook & Crisp Basket" in the pot of Ninja Foodi.
4. Close the Ninja Foodi with crisping lid and select "Air Crisp".
5. Press "Start/Stop" to begin and set the temperature to 355 degrees F.
6. Set the time for 5 minutes to preheat.
7. Now, place the salmon fillets into "Cook & Crisp Basket".
8. Close the Ninja Foodi with crisping lid and select "Air Crisp".
9. Set the temperature to 355 degrees F for 13 minutes.
10. Press "Start/Stop" to begin. After 8 minutes, flip the salmon fillets and coat with reserved marinade.
11. Open the lid and serve.
- **Nutrition Info:** Calories: 299; Carbohydrates: 37.4g; Protein: 24.1g; Fat: 7g; Sugar: 35.3g; Sodium: 1600mg; Fiber: 0.3g

128.Family Feast Shrimp

Servings: 4
Cooking Time: 20 Minutes
Ingredients:
- 1 lb. shrimp, peeled and deveined
- Salt and freshly ground black pepper, to taste
- 8-oz. coconut milk
- ½ C. panko breadcrumbs
- ½ tsp. cayenne pepper

Directions:
1. In a shallow dish, mix together the coconut milk, salt and black pepper.
2. In another shallow dish, mix together breadcrumbs, cayenne pepper, salt and black pepper.
3. Dip the shrimp in coconut milk mixture and then coat with the breadcrumbs mixture. Arrange the "Cook & Crisp Basket" in the pot of Ninja Foodi.
4. Close the Ninja Foodi with crisping lid and select "Air Crisp".
5. Press "Start/Stop" to begin and set the temperature to 350 degrees F.
6. Set the time for 5 minutes to preheat.
7. Now, place the shrimp into "Cook & Crisp Basket". Close the Ninja Foodi with crisping lid and select "Air Crisp".
8. Set the temperature to 350 degrees F for 20 minutes.
9. Press "Start/Stop" to begin. Open the lid and serve.
- **Nutrition Info:** Calories: 301; Carbohydrates: 12.5g; Protein: 28.2g; Fat: 15.7g; Sugar: 2.2g; Sodium: 393mg; Fiber: 2.3g

129.Mexican Swordfish

Servings: 4 Servings
Cooking Time: 8 Minutes
Ingredients:
- 4 Swordfish Steaks
- ½ cup water
- 1 cup chopped tomatoes
- ½ cup chopped onion
- 1 tbsp lime juice
- 1 jalapeno, seeds removed, chopped
- ½ tsp salt

- ¼ tsp ground black pepper

Directions:
1. Place the swordfish in the Ninja Foodi pot and add all the ingredients to the bowl.
2. Close the pressure seal lid and set the steamer valve to seal.
3. Cook on high pressure for 8 minutes then do a quick pressure release. Serve the swordfish while hot.
- **Nutrition Info:** Calories: 177g, Carbohydrates: 8g, Protein: 23g, Fat: 6g, Sugar: 5g, Sodium: 684

130.French Salmon Meal

Servings: 6
Cooking Time: 5 Hours 55 Minutes
Ingredients:
- ¾ C. green lentils
- 1 C. carrot, peeled and chopped
- 2 C. chicken broth
- Salt and freshly ground black pepper, to taste
- 6 (4-oz.) skinless, boneless salmon fillets

Directions:
1. In the pot of Ninja Foodi, place all ingredients except the salmon and stir to combine.
2. Close the crisping lid and select "Slow Cooker".
3. Set on "High" for about 5-5½ hours
4. Press "Start/Stop" to begin.
5. Open the lid and arrange a large parchment paper over lentil mixture.
6. Season the salmon fillets with salt and black pepper evenly.
7. Arrange the salmon fillets over parchment paper in a single layer.
8. Close the crisping lid and select "Slow Cooker".
9. Set on "High" for about 25 minutes.
10. Press "Start/Stop" to begin.
11. Open the lid and serve the salmon fillets with lentil mixture.
- **Nutrition Info:** Calories: 247; Carbohydrates: 16.5g; Protein: 33.3g; Fat: 4.8g; Sugar: 1.6g; Sodium: 336mg; Fiber: 7.8g

131.Salmon Stew

Servings: 3
Cooking Time: 16 Minutes
Ingredients:
- 1 c. homemade fish broth
- Salt and black pepper
- 1 chopped onion
- 1 lb. salmon fillet, cubed
- 1 tbsp. butter

Directions:
1. Season the salmon fillets with salt and black pepper.
2. Press "Sauté" on Ninja Foodi and add butter and onions.
3. Sauté for about 3 minutes and add salmon and fish broth.
4. Lock the lid and set the Ninja Foodi to "Pressure" for about 8 minutes.
5. Release the pressure naturally and dish out to serve hot.
- **Nutrition Info:** 272 calories, 14.2g fat, 4.4g carbs, 32.1g protein

132.Bok Choy On Ginger-sesame Salmon

Servings: 2
Cooking Time: 6 Minutes
Ingredients:
- 1 tablespoon toasted sesame oil
- 1 tablespoons rice vinegar
- 2 tablespoons sear button sugar
- 1/2 cup shoyu (soy sauce)
- 1 garlic clove, pressed
- 1 tablespoon freshly grated ginger
- 1 tablespoon toasted sesame seed
- 2 green onions, sliced reserve some for garnish
- 2 7-oz salmon filet
- 2 baby bok choy washed well
- 1 teaspoon miso paste mixed with a 1/2 cup of water

Directions:
1. On a loaf pan that fits inside your Ninja Foodi, place salmon with skin side down.
2. In a small bowl whisk well sesame oil, rice vinegar, sear button sugar, shoyu, garlic, ginger, and sesame seed. Pour over salmon.

3. Place half of sliced green onions over salmon. Securely cover pan with foil.
4. On a separate loaf pan, place bok choy. In a small bowl, whisk well water and miso paste. Pour over bok choy and seal pan securely with foil.
5. Add water to Ninja Foodi and place trivet. Place pan of salmon side by side the bok choy pan on trivet.
6. Install pressure lid. Close Ninja Foodi, press manual button, choose high settings, and set time to 6 minutes.
7. Once done cooking, do a quick release. Serve and enjoy.
- **Nutrition Info:** Calories: 609; carbohydrates: 30.4g; protein: 56.0g; fat: 29.2g

133.Lemon Cod

Servings: 2 Servings
Cooking Time: 5 Minutes
Ingredients:
- ½ cup water
- 2 Tbsp butter
- 1/3 cup lemon juice
- 1 pound cod filets
- ½ tsp paprika

Directions:
1. Add all the ingredients into the cook and crisp basket and place the basket inside the Ninja Foodi.
2. Place the pressure cooker lid on top of the pot and close the pressure valve to the seal position. Set the pressure cooker function to high heat and set the timer for 3 minutes.
3. Once the coking cycle is complete, release the pressure quickly by carefully opening the steamer valve. Enjoy while hot
- **Nutrition Info:** Calories: 492g, Carbohydrates: 3g, Protein: 82g, Fat: 15g, Sugar: 1g, Sodium: 335mg

134.Mesmerizing Salmon Loaf

Servings: 6
Cooking Time: 6 Hours 10 Mins
Ingredients:
- 2 slightly beaten eggs
- 1 c. chicken broth

- ¼ c. shredded cheddar cheese
- 2 c. stuffing croutons, seasoned
- 7 oz. drained salmon, skinless and boneless

Directions:
1. Mix all the ingredients except salmon in a bowl then add salmon and combine it well
2. Spray the inside of the Ninja Foodi with cooking spray
3. Make it into a loaf shape
4. Cook for 4-6 hours on low heat
5. Serve and enjoy!
- **Nutrition Info:** 220 calories, 5g fat, 13g carbs, 20g protein

135.Salmon-pesto Over Pasta

Servings: 2
Cooking Time: 10 Minutes
Ingredients:
- 4 ounces dry pasta
- 1 cup water
- 3-ounces smoked salmon, broken up in bite sized pieces
- 1/4 lemon
- Salt and pepper
- 1/2 teaspoon grated lemon zest
- 1/2 teaspoon lemon juice
- 2 tbsp heavy cream
- Pesto-spinach sauce ingredients:
- 1 tbsp walnuts
- 1 clove garlic
- 1 cup packed baby spinach
- 1 ½ tbsp olive oil
- 1/4 cup freshly grated parmesan + more for serving/garnish
- Kosher salt and black pepper to taste
- 1 tsp grated lemon zest
- 1/4 cup heavy cream

Directions:
1. Make the sauce in blender by pulsing garlic and walnuts until chopped. Add ¼ tsp pepper, ¼ tsp salt, ½ cup parmesan, oil, and 2/3s of spinach. Puree until smooth.
2. Add butter, water, and pasta in Ninja Foodi.
3. Install pressure lid. Close Ninja Foodi, press pressure button, choose high settings, and set time to 4 minutes.
4. Once done cooking, do a quick release. Press stop and then press sauté.

5. Stir in remaining parmesan, remaining spinach, sauce, lemon juice, lemon zest, heavy cream, and smoked salmon. Mix well and sauté for 5 minutes.
6. Serve and enjoy.
- **Nutrition Info:** Calories: 465; carbohydrates: 31.0g; protein: 20.1g; fat: 29.0g

136.Green Chili Mahi-mahi Fillets

Servings: 2
Cooking Time: 10 Minutes
Ingredients:
- ¼ c. homemade green chili enchilada sauce
- 2 thawed Mahi-Mahi fillets
- 2 tbsps. butter
- Salt and pepper
- 1 c. water

Directions:
1. Pour 1 cup of water into the Ninja Foodi and set a steamer rack.
2. Grease the bottom of each mahi-mahi fillet with 1 tablespoon of butter, spreading the butter from end to end – this will prevent the fish from sticking to the rack.
3. Put the fillets on the rack. Spread 1/4 cup of enchilada sauce between each fillet using a pastry brush – cover them well.
4. Top with more enchilada sauce, if desired. Season fillets with salt and pepper. Lock the lid and close the steam valve. Press "PRESSURE", set the pressure to HIGH, and set the timer for 5 minutes.
5. When the timer beeps, quickly release the pressure and transfer the fillets into serving plates. Serve.
- **Nutrition Info:** 120 calories, 2g fat, 5g carbs, 10g protein

137.Bbq Shrimp

Servings: 4 Servings
Cooking Time: 12 Minutes
Ingredients:
- 1 ½ pounds Shrimp, deveined and peeled
- 1 Tbsp olive oil
- 1 tsp ground paprika
- ¼ tsp salt
- ¼ tsp ground black pepper

- 1 onion, chopped
- ¼ cup hot sauce
- 1 tsp stevia
- ¼ cup water
- 2 Tbsp vinegar

Directions:
1. Turn the Ninja Foodi on to saute and add the olive oil. Once hot, add the shrimp and sear on each side for 2 minutes.
2. Sprinkle the salt and pepper on the shrimp and then add all the remaining ingredients to the pot.
3. Cover the Foodi and use the pressure cooker function to cook the shrimp for 8 minutes under high heat pressure.
4. Release the pressure using a natural steam and serve warm or chilled
- **Nutrition Info:** Calories: 207g, Carbohydrates: 1g, Protein: 36g, Fat: 6g, Sugar: 2g, Sodium: 3633mg

138.Miso Glazed Salmon

Servings: 4
Cooking Time: 9 Minutes
Ingredients:
- 4 (4-oz.) (1-inch thick) frozen skinless salmon fillets
- Salt, to taste
- 2 tbsp. butter, softened
- 2 tbsp. red miso paste
- 2 heads baby bok choy, stems on, cut in half

Directions:
1. In the pot of Ninja Foodi, place ½ C. of water. In the pot, arrange the reversible rack in higher position. Season the salmon fillets with salt evenly.
2. Place the salmon fillets over the rack. Cover the Ninja Foodi with the pressure lid and place the pressure valve to "Seal" position.
3. Select "Pressure" and set to "High" for about 2 minutes.
4. Press "Start/Stop" to begin. Switch the valve to "Vent" and do a "Quick" release.
5. Meanwhile, spray the bok choy with cooking spray evenly.
6. In a bowl, add the butter and miso paste and mix well. Once all the pressure is released, open the lid. With paper towels,

pat dry the salmon fillets and then, coat them with butter mixture evenly.

7. Arrange the bok choy around the salmon fillets,
8. Now, close the Ninja Foodi with crisping lid and select "Broil".
9. Set time to 7 minutes and select "Start/Stop" to begin.
10. Open the lid and serve the salmon fillets alongside the bok choy.
- **Nutrition Info:** Calories: 210; Carbohydrates: 9g; Protein: 24.2g; Fat: 9g; Sugar: 5.5g; Sodium: 897mg; Fiber: 3.4g

139.Butter Shrimp

Servings: 4 Servings
Cooking Time: 12 Minutes
Ingredients:
- 2 pounds shrimp, deveined and peeled
- 2 Tbsp Butter
- 1 tsp chili powder
- 1 tsp garlic powder
- ½ tsp ground black pepper
- ¼ cup parmesan cheese

Directions:
1. Place the shrimp and butter in the pot and press saute. Sear both sides of the shrimp for 2 minutes.
2. Sprinkle the chili powder, garlic powder and ground black pepper on the shrimp and mix. Sprinkle the cheese over the shrimp and place the air crisp lid on top.
3. Use the roast function set to 375 to cook the shrimp for 10 more minutes. Serve hot.
- **Nutrition Info:** Calories: 293, Carbohydrates: 2g, Protein: 66g, Fat: 13g, Sugar: 0g, Sodium: 1386 mg

140.Eggs 'n Smoked Ramekin

Servings: 2
Cooking Time: 4 Minutes
Ingredients:
- 2 eggs
- 2 slices of smoked salmon
- 2 slices of cheese
- 2 fresh basil leaves for garnish
- Olive oil

Directions:

1. Add a cup of water in Ninja Foodi and place trivet on bottom.
2. Lightly grease each ramekin with a drop of olive oil each. Spread well.
3. Crack an egg in each ramekin. Place a slice of cheese, a slice of smoked salmon, and basil leaf in each ramekin.
4. Cover each ramekin with foil and place on trivet.
5. Install pressure lid. Close Ninja Foodi, press manual button, choose low settings, and set time to 4 minutes.
6. Once done cooking, do a quick release.
7. Serve and enjoy.
- **Nutrition Info:** Calories: 239; carbohydrates: 0.9g; protein: 17.5g; fat: 18.3g

141.Seafood Gumbo New Orleans Style

Servings: 2
Cooking Time: 20 Minutes
Ingredients:
- 1 sea bass filet patted dry and cut into 2" chunks
- 1 tablespoon ghee or avocado oil
- 1 tablespoon Cajun seasoning
- 1 small yellow onion diced
- 1 small bell pepper diced
- 1 celery rib diced
- 2 roma tomatoes diced
- 1 tbsp tomato paste
- 1 bay leaf
- 1/2 cup bone broth
- ¾-pound medium to large raw shrimp deveined
- Sea salt to taste
- Black pepper to taste

Directions:
1. Press sauté button and heat oil.
2. Season fish chunks with pepper, salt, and half of Cajun seasoning. Once oil is hot, sear fish chunks for 3 minutes per side and gently transfer to a plate.
3. Stir in remaining Cajun seasoning, celery, and onions. Sauté for 2 minutes. Press stop.
4. Stir in bone broth, bay leaves, tomato paste, and diced tomatoes. Mix well. Add back fish.

Install pressure lid and place valve to vent position.

5. Close Ninja Foodi, press pressure cook button, choose high settings, and set time to 5 minutes.
6. Once done cooking, do a quick release. Stir in shrimps. Cover and let it sit for 5 minutes. Open and mix well.
7. Serve and enjoy.
- **Nutrition Info:** Calories: 357; carbohydrates: 14.8g; protein: 45.9g; fat: 12.6g

142.Wine Braised Salmon

Servings: 6
Cooking Time: 1 Hour
Ingredients:
- 1½ C. chicken broth
- ½ C. white wine
- 1 shallot, sliced thinly
- 4 (4-oz.) salmon fillets
- Salt and freshly ground black pepper, to taste

Directions:
1. In the pot of Ninja Foodi, mix together broth, shallot and lemon.
2. Arrange salmon fillets on top, skin side down and sprinkle with salt and black pepper.
3. Close the crisping lid and select "Slow Cooker".
4. Set on "Low" for about 45-60 minutes.
5. Press "Start/Stop" to begin.
6. Open the lid and serve hot.
- **Nutrition Info:** Calories: 192; Carbohydrates: 1.9g; Protein: 24g; Fat: 7.5g; Sugar: 0.5g; Sodium: 377mg; Fiber: 0g

143.Easy Veggie-salmon Bake

Servings: 2
Cooking Time: 20 Minutes
Ingredients:
- 1 cup chicken broth
- 1 cup milk
- 1 salmon filet
- 2 tbsp olive oil
- Ground pepper to taste
- 1 tsp minced garlic

- 1 cup frozen vegetables
- 1/2 can of cream of celery soup
- ¼ tsp dill
- ¼ tsp cilantro
- 1 tsp Italian spice
- 1 tsp poultry seasoning
- 1 tbsp ground parmesan

Directions:
1. Press sauté button and heat oil.
2. Add the salmon and cook until white on both sides and defrosted enough to split apart, around 2 minutes per side.
3. Add the garlic and just stir into the oil then deglaze the pot with the broth for 3 minutes.
4. Add the spices, milk, vegetables, noodles and stir.
5. Add the cream of celery soup on top and just gently stir so it is mixed in enough on top to not be clumpy.
6. Install pressure lid. Close Ninja Foodi, press pressure cook button, choose high settings, and set time to 8 minutes.
7. Once done cooking, do a quick release.
8. Serve and enjoy with a sprinkle of parmesan.
- **Nutrition Info:** Calories: 616; carbohydrates: 28.7g; protein: 51.8g; fat: 32.6g

144.Spicy Shrimp Soup

Servings: 4 Servings
Cooking Time: 10 Minutes
Ingredients:
- 1 pound shrimp, deveined
- 6 cups chicken broth
- 2 cloves of garlic, chopped
- 1 carrot, chopped
- 2 Bell peppers, chopped
- 2 celery stalks, chopped
- ½ white onion, chopped
- ¼ tsp salt
- ½ tsp cayenne pepper
- 1/8 tsp ground black pepper

Directions:
1. Add all the ingredients to the pot and place the pressure cooker lid on the Ninja Foodi.
2. Cook on high pressure for 10 minutes. Do a quick steam release and remove the lid.

3. Remove the chicken from the pot and shred the chicken using two forks.
4. Serve while hot or freeze to use at a later date.
- **Nutrition Info:** Calories: 150g, Carbohydrates: 2g, Protein: 36g, Fat: 0g, Sugar: 2g, Sodium: 438mg

145.Buffalo Fish

Servings: 6
Cooking Time: 21 Minutes
Ingredients:
- 6 tbsps. butter
- ¾ c. Franks red hot sauce
- 6 fish fillets
- Salt and black pepper
- 2 tsps. garlic powder

Directions:
1. Press "Sauté" on Ninja Foodi and add butter and fish fillets.
2. Sauté for about 3 minutes and add salt, black pepper and garlic powder.
3. Press "Bake/Roast" and bake for about 8 minutes at 340 degrees F.
4. Dish out in a serving platter and serve hot.
- **Nutrition Info:** 317 calories, 22.7g fat, 16.4g carbs, 13.6g protein

146.Salmon And Asparagus

Servings: 2 Servings
Cooking Time: 5 Minutes
Ingredients:
- ½ cup water
- 2 Tbsp butter
- 1 lemon, sliced
- 1 pound Salmon, de boned
- ½ ground black pepper
- 1 bunch asparagus, about ½ pound

Directions:
1. Add all the ingredients into the cook and crisp basket, with the asparagus on the bottom, the lemon slices layered on the salmon, and place the basket inside the Ninja Foodi.
2. Place the pressure cooker lid on top of the pot and close the pressure valve to the seal position. Set the pressure cooker function to high heat and set the timer for 3 minutes.

3. Once the cooking cycle is complete, release the pressure quickly by carefully opening the steamer valve. Enjoy while hot
- **Nutrition Info:** Calories: 342g, Carbohydrates: 13g, Protein: 46g, Fat: 14g, Sugar: 4g, Sodium: 568mg

147.Lemon Pepper Salmon

Servings: 2 Servings
Cooking Time: 5 Minutes
Ingredients:
- ½ cup water
- 2 Tbsp butter
- 1/3 cup lemon juice
- 1 pound Salmon, de boned
- ½ ground black pepper

Directions:
1. Add all the ingredients into the cook and crisp basket and place the basket inside the Ninja Foodi.
2. Place the pressure cooker lid on top of the pot and close the pressure valve to the seal position. Set the pressure cooker function to high heat and set the timer for 3 minutes.
3. Once the coking cycle is complete, release the pressure quickly by carefully opening the steamer valve. Enjoy while hot
- **Nutrition Info:** Calories: 314g, Carbohydrates: 8g, Protein: 42g, Fat: 14g, Sugar: 1g, Sodium: 565g

148.Sweet 'n Spicy Mahi-mahi

Servings: 2
Cooking Time: 10 Minutes
Ingredients:
- 2 6-oz mahi-mahi fillets
- Salt, to taste
- Black pepper, to taste
- 1-2 cloves garlic, minced or crushed
- 1" piece ginger, finely grated
- ½ lime, juiced
- 2 tablespoons honey
- 1 tablespoon nanami togarashi
- 2 tablespoons sriracha
- 1 tablespoon orange juice

Directions:
1. In a heatproof dish that fits inside the Ninja Foodi, mix well orange juice, sriracha,

nanami togarashi, honey lime juice, ginger, and garlic.
2. Season mahi-mahi with pepper and salt. Place in bowl of sauce and cover well in sauce. Seal dish securely with foil.
3. Install pressure lid and place valve to vent position.
4. Add a cup of water in Ninja Foodi, place trivet, and add dish of mahi-mahi on trivet.
5. Close Ninja Foodi, press steam button and set time to 10 minutes.
6. Once done cooking, do a quick release.
7. Serve and enjoy.
- **Nutrition Info:** Calories: 200; carbohydrates: 20.1g; protein: 28.1g; fat: 0.8g

149.Chili Lime Salmon

Servings: 2 Servings
Cooking Time: 5 Minutes
Ingredients:
- ½ cup water
- 2 Tbsp butter
- 1/3 cup lime juice
- 1 pound Salmon, de boned
- ½ ground chili powder

Directions:
1. Add the salmon into the cook and crisp basket and place the basket inside the Ninja Foodi.
2. Sprinkle the chili powder over the top of the salmon and then add the water, butter and lime juice around the filets.
3. Place the pressure cooker lid on top of the pot and close the pressure valve to the seal position. Set the pressure cooker function to high heat and set the timer for 3 minutes.
4. Once the cooking cycle is complete, release the pressure quickly by carefully opening the steamer valve. Enjoy while hot
- **Nutrition Info:** Calories: 349g, Carbohydrates: 8g, Protein: 44g, Fat: 17g, Sugar: 1g, Sodium: 566g

150.Veggie Fish Soup

Servings: 4 Servings
Cooking Time: 10 Minutes
Ingredients:

- 1 pound cod
- 6 cups chicken broth
- 2 cloves of garlic, chopped
- 1 carrot, chopped
- 1 Bell pepper, chopped
- 1 sweet potato, peeled, diced
- 2 celery stalks, chopped
- ½ white onion, chopped
- ¼ tsp salt
- 1/8 tsp ground black pepper
- ¼ cup shredded cheddar cheese

Directions:
1. Add all the ingredients to the pot and place the pressure cooker lid on the Ninja Foodi.
2. Cook on high pressure for 10 minutes. Do a quick steam release and remove the lid.
3. Remove the chicken from the pot and shred the chicken using two forks.
4. Serve while hot or freeze to use at a later date.
- **Nutrition Info:** Calories: 250g, Carbohydrates: 4g, Protein: 36g, Fat: 0g, Sugar: 2g, Sodium: 438mg

151.Rosemary Scallops

Servings: 6
Cooking Time: 6 Minutes
Ingredients:
- ½ C. butter
- 4 garlic cloves, minced
- 2 tbsp. fresh rosemary, chopped
- 2 lb. sea scallops
- Salt and freshly ground black pepper, to taste

Directions:
1. Select "Sauté/Sear" setting of Ninja Foodi and place the butter into the pot.
2. Press "Start/Stop" to begin and heat for about 2-3 minutes.
3. Add the garlic and rosemary and cook, uncovered for about 1 minute.
4. Stir in the scallops, salt and black pepper and cook for about 2 minutes.
5. Press "Start/Stop" to stop the cooking.
6. Now, close the Ninja Foodi with crisping lid and select "Air Crisp".
7. Set the temperature to 350 degrees F for 3 minutes.

8. Press "Start/Stop" to begin. Open the lid and serve.
- **Nutrition Info:** Calories: 275; Carbohydrates: 4.9g; Protein: 25.7g; Fat: 16.7g; Sugar: 0g; Sodium: 380mg; Fiber: 0.5g

152.Salmon With Orange-ginger Sauce

Servings: 2
Cooking Time: 15 Minutes
Ingredients:
- 1-pound salmon
- 1 tablespoon dark soy sauce
- 2 teaspoons minced ginger
- 1 teaspoon minced garlic
- 1 teaspoon salt
- 1 1/2 tsp ground pepper
- 2 tablespoons low sugar marmalade

Directions:
1. In a heatproof pan that fits inside your Ninja Foodi, add salmon.
2. Mix all the sauce ingredients and pour over the salmon. Allow to marinate for 15-30 minutes. Cover pan with foil securely.
3. Put 2 cups of water in Ninja Foodi and add trivet.
4. Place the pan of salmon on trivet.
5. Install pressure lid. Close Ninja Foodi, press pressure button, choose low settings, and set time to 5 minutes.
6. Once done cooking, do a quick release.
7. Serve and enjoy.
- **Nutrition Info:** Calories: 177; carbohydrates: 8.8g; protein: 24.0g; fat: 5.0g

153.Coconut Curry Fish

Servings: 2
Cooking Time: 15 Minutes
Ingredients:
- 1-lb fish steaks or fillets, rinsed and cut into bite-size pieces
- 1 tomato, chopped
- 1 green chiles, sliced into strips
- 1 small onions, sliced into strips
- 2 garlic cloves, squeezed
- 1/2 tbsp freshly grated ginger
- 2 bay laurel leaves
- 1 tsp ground coriander

- 1 tsp ground cumin
- ½ tsp ground turmeric
- ½ tsp chili powder
- ½ tsp ground fenugreek
- 1 cup unsweetened coconut milk
- Salt to taste

Directions:
1. Press sauté button and heat oil. Add garlic, sauté for a minute. Stir in ginger and onions. Sauté for 5 minutes. Stir in bay leaves, fenugreek, chili powder, turmeric, cumin, and coriander. Cook for a minute.
2. Add coconut milk and deglaze pot.
3. Stir in tomatoes and green chilies. Mix well.
4. Add fish and mix well. Install pressure lid and place valve to vent position.
5. Close Ninja Foodi, press pressure cook button, choose low settings, and set time to 5 minutes.
6. Once done cooking, do a quick release. Adjust seasoning to taste.
7. Serve and enjoy.
- **Nutrition Info:** Calories: 434; carbohydrates: 11.7g; protein: 29.7g; fat: 29.8g

154.Coconut Curry Sea Bass

Servings: 2
Cooking Time: 3 Minutes
Ingredients:
- 1 (14.5 ounce) can coconut milk
- Juice of 1 lime
- 1 tablespoon red curry paste
- 1 teaspoon fish sauce
- 1 teaspoon coconut aminos
- 1 teaspoon honey
- 2 teaspoons sriracha
- 2 cloves garlic, minced
- 1 teaspoon ground turmeric
- 1 teaspoon ground ginger
- 1/2 teaspoon sea salt
- 1/2 teaspoon white pepper
- 1-pound sea bass, cut into 1" cubes
- 1/4 cup chopped fresh cilantro
- 2 lime wedges

Directions:
1. Whisk well pepper, salt, ginger, turmeric, garlic, sriracha, honey, coconut aminos, fish

sauce, red curry paste, lime juice, and coconut milk in a large bowl.
2. Place fish in pot and pour coconut milk mixture over it.
3. Install pressure lid. Close Ninja Foodi, press pressure button, choose high settings, and set time to 3 minutes.
4. Once done cooking, do a quick release.
5. Serve and enjoy with equal amounts of lime wedge and cilantro.
- **Nutrition Info:** Calories: 749; carbohydrates: 16.6g; protein: 58.0g; fat: 50.0g

155.Fancy "rich" Guy Smoked Lobster

Servings: 4
Cooking Time: 35 Minutes
Ingredients:
- 6 Lobster Tails
- 4 garlic cloves
- ¼ c. butter

Directions:
1. Preheat the Ninja Foodi to 400 degrees F at first
2. Open the lobster tails gently by using kitchen scissors
3. Remove the lobster meat gently from the shells but keep it inside the shells
4. Take a plate and place it
5. Add some butter in a pan and allow it melt
6. Put some garlic cloves in it and heat it over medium-low heat
7. Pour the garlic butter mixture all over the lobster tail meat
8. Let the fryer to broil the lobster at 130 degrees F
9. Remove the lobster meat from Ninja Foodi and set aside
10. Use a fork to pull out the lobster meat from the shells entirely
11. Pour some garlic butter over it if needed
- **Nutrition Info:** 160 calories, 1g fat, 3g carbs, 20g protein

156.Pepper Crusted Tuna

Servings: 2 Servings
Cooking Time: 5 Minutes
Ingredients:

- ½ cup water
- 2 Tbsp butter
- 1/3 cup lemon juice
- 1 pound Tuna Filets
- T tsp black peppercorns, crushed

Directions:
1. Rub the tuna with the black pepper and then place in the air crisper basket.
2. Place the basket into the Ninja Foodi.
3. Sprinkle the chili powder over the top of the salmon and then add the butter and lemon juice around the filets.
4. Place the pressure cooker lid on top of the pot and close the pressure valve to the seal position. Set the pressure cooker function to high heat and set the timer for 3 minutes.
5. Once the cooking cycle is complete, release the pressure quickly by carefully opening the steamer valve. Enjoy while hot
- **Nutrition Info:** Calories: 564g, Carbohydrates: 3g, Protein: 52g, Fat: 39g, Sugar: 1g, Sodium: 85mg

157.Buttered Scallops

Servings: 6
Cooking Time: 25 Minutes
Ingredients:
- 4 minced garlic cloves
- 4 tbsps. freshly chopped rosemary,
- 2 lbs. sea scallops
- ½ c. butter
- Salt and black pepper

Directions:
1. Press "Sauté" on Ninja Foodi and add butter, rosemary and garlic.
2. Sauté for about 1 minute and add sea scallops, salt and black pepper.
3. Sauté for about 2 minutes and press "Air Crisp" at 350 degrees F.
4. Set the timer for about 3 minutes and dish out to serve.
- **Nutrition Info:** 279 calories, 16.8g fat, 5.7g carbs, 25.8g protein

158.Salsa Tuna Steaks

Servings: 4 Servings
Cooking Time: 10 Minutes
Ingredients:

- 4 Tuna Steaks, about 2 pounds
- ½ cup water
- 1 cup chopped tomatoes
- ½ cup chopped onion
- 1 tbsp lemon juice
- ½ tsp salt
- ¼ tsp ground black pepper

Directions:

1. Place the tuna in the Ninja Foodi pot and add all the ingredients to the bowl.
2. Close the pressure seal lid and set the steamer valve to seal.
3. Cook on high pressure for 8 minutes then do a quick pressure release. Serve the tuna while hot.
- **Nutrition Info:** Calories: 165g, Carbohydrates: 4g, Protein: 24g, Fat: 3g, Sugar: 3g, Sodium: 583 mg

159.Buttered Halibut

Servings: 4
Cooking Time: 30 Minutes
Ingredients:

- 1 lb. halibut fillets
- 2 tbsp. ginger-garlic paste
- Salt and freshly ground black pepper, to taste
- 3 green chilies, chopped
- ¾ C. butter, chopped

Directions:

1. Select "Bake/Roast" of Ninja Foodi and set the temperature to 360 degrees F.
2. Press "Start/Stop" to begin and preheat the Ninja Foodi for about 10 minutes.
3. Coat the halibut fillets with ginger-garlic paste and then, season with salt and black pepper.
4. In the pot of Ninja Foodi, place the halibut fillets and top with green chilies, followed by the butter.

5. Close the Ninja Foodi with crisping lid and set the time for 30 minutes.
6. Press "Start/Stop" to begin. Open the lid and serve.
- **Nutrition Info:** Calories: 517; Carbohydrates: 2.4g; Protein: 31.5g; Fat: 41.6g; Sugar: 0.2g; Sodium: 364mg; Fiber: 0.1g

160.Tomato-basil Dressed Tilapia

Servings: 2
Cooking Time: 4 Minutes
Ingredients:

- 2 (4 oz) tilapia fillets
- Salt and pepper
- 2 roma tomatoes, diced
- 2 minced garlic cloves
- 1/4 cup chopped basil (fresh)
- 1 tbsp olive oil
- 1/4 tsp salt
- 1/8 tsp pepper
- 1 tbsp Balsamic vinegar (optional)

Directions:

1. Add a cup of water in Ninja Foodi, place steamer basket, and add tilapia in basket. Season with pepper and salt.
2. Install pressure lid and place valve to vent position.
3. Close Ninja Foodi, press steam button, and set time to 2 minutes.
4. Meanwhile, in a medium bowl toss well to mix pepper, salt, olive oil, basil, garlic, and tomatoes. If desired, you can add a tablespoon of balsamic vinegar. Mix well.
5. Once done cooking, do a quick release.
6. Serve and enjoy with the basil-tomato dressing.
- **Nutrition Info:** Calories: 196; carbohydrates: 2.0g; protein: 20.0g; fat: 12.0g

SOUPS & STEWS

161.Creamy Chicken & Mushroom Soup

Servings: 6 Servings
Cooking Time: 15 Minutes
Ingredients:
- 6 chicken thighs, boneless, skinless and cut into 1-inch pieces
- 4 cups chicken broth
- 1 cup cremini mushrooms, sliced thin
- 3 carrots, peeled and chopped fine
- 2 stalks celery, chopped fine
- 1 onion, chopped fine
- ½ cup half-and-half
- ¼ cup flour
- 3 cloves garlic, chopped fine
- 2 tablespoons butter
- 2 tablespoons fresh parsley, chopped
- 1 tablespoon olive oil
- ½ teaspoon thyme
- 1 sprig rosemary
- 1 bay leaf
- Salt & pepper

Directions:
1. Add the olive oil to the pot and set to sauté on medium heat. Sprinkle the chicken with salt and pepper and add to the pot. Cook till brown, about 2-3 minutes, set aside.
2. Add the butter and let it melt. Once melted, add the vegetables and cook till tender, about 3-4 minutes. Stir in thyme and cook 1 minute more.
3. Stir in flour till lightly browned, about 1 minute. Add the broth, bay leaf, rosemary and chicken and cook, stirring constantly, till soup thickens, about 4-5 minutes.
4. Stir in the half-and-half and continue cooking till heated through, 1-2 minutes. Discard bay leaf and rosemary sprig. Serve immediately.

162.Autumn Stew

Servings: 4 -6 Servings
Cooking Time: 8 Hours
Ingredients:
- 1 pound smoked sausage, sliced, not too thin
- 4 potatoes, peeled and quartered
- 3 carrots, peeled and chopped
- 3 stalks celery, sliced
- 2-3 turnips, peeled and cubed
- 1 small cabbage, cut into chunks
- 1 large can of tomatoes, diced
- 1 teaspoon sage
- 1 teaspoon oregano
- 1 teaspoon basil
- ½ teaspoon thyme
- ½ teaspoon rosemary
- Salt & pepper

Directions:
1. Layer the ingredients in the cooking pot; carrots, turnips, celery, potatoes and cabbage, sprinkling each layer with a little of the herbs, salt and pepper.
2. Spread tomatoes, with liquid, over cabbage and top with sausage. Sprinkle more seasonings on top.
3. Secure the lid and select slow cooking function. The stew will take 7-8 hours on low or 4-5 on high heat. The stew is done with vegetables are tender. Stir well before serving.

163.Duck Ale Chili

Servings: 6 Servings
Cooking Time: 45 Minutes
Ingredients:
- 1 ½ pound duck breast
- 1 large can fire roasted tomatoes, diced
- 1 can kidney beans, rinsed and drained
- 1 can great northern beans, rinsed and drained
- 1 bottle brown ale
- 1 small can tomato paste
- 1 cup white onion, chopped fine
- 5 cloves garlic, chopped fine
- 2 tablespoons chili powder
- 1 tablespoon Worcestershire
- 1 tablespoon oregano
- 2 teaspoons cumin
- 1 teaspoon salt
- 1 teaspoon ground black pepper
- 1 teaspoon smoked paprika

- 1 teaspoon onion powder
- 1 teaspoon red pepper flakes
- ½ teaspoon cayenne pepper
- Garnishes:
- 1 cup mozzarella cheese, grated
- ½ cup chopped cilantro

Directions:

1. Score the fat on the duck and sprinkle with salt. Place, fat side down, in the cooking pot.
2. Select sauté on medium heat and sear the duck till golden brown and most of the fat has been rendered. Transfer duck to a plate.
3. Add the onions and cook till they soften, about 5 minutes. Add the duck back to the pot along with remaining ingredients.
4. Secure the lid and set to pressure cooking on high. Set the timer for 30 minutes. When the timer goes off, use manual release to remove the lid.
5. Remove the duck and shred with two forks. Return it to the pot and stir well.
6. Ladle into bowl and top with garnishes before serving.

164. Poblano Beef Stew

Servings: 4 – 6 Servings
Cooking Time: 1 Hour
Ingredients:

- 1 ½ pounds beef chuck roast, cut into 1-inch cubes
- 4 cups beef broth
- 15 ounce can fire roasted tomatoes
- 3 large poblano peppers
- 2 potatoes, cut into 1-inch cubes
- 1 onion, chopped
- 2-3 tablespoons cilantro, chopped
- 1 tablespoon olive oil
- 1 tablespoon garlic, chopped fine
- 1 ½ teaspoon ground cumin
- 1 teaspoon oregano

Directions:

1. Place the poblano chilies in the cooker. Add the Tender Crisp lid and set to broil. Cook the chilies 5-7 minutes, turning a couple of times, till skin is charred. Place them in a bowl and cover with foil. Let sit 10 minutes, then remove the skin. Remove the ribs and seeds and cut into 1-inch pieces.

2. Add the oil to the pot and set to sauté on med-high heat. Sprinkle the beef with salt and pepper and add to the pot, in batches. Cook the beef till no longer pink. Remove and set aside.
3. Add the onions and cook till they are translucent, about 3-5 minutes. Add the garlic and cook another 30 seconds. Add remaining ingredients except the potatoes and cilantro and stir to combine.
4. Secure the lid and set to pressure cooking on high. Set the timer for 40 minutes. When the timer goes off use quick release to remove the lid.
5. Add the potatoes and pressure cook on high another 8-10 minutes. Use quick release again. Stir and ladle into bowls. Top with chopped cilantro before serving.

165. Filling Cauli-squash Chowder

Servings: 2
Cooking Time: 12 Minutes
Ingredients:

- 1 tablespoon oil
- 1/2 onion, diced
- 1 clove garlic, minced
- 1/2-pound frozen cauliflower
- 1/2-pound frozen butternut squash
- 1 cup vegetable broth
- 1/2 teaspoon paprika
- 1/2 teaspoon dried thyme
- Salt and pepper to taste
- 1/4 cup half-and-half

Directions:

1. Press the sauté button on the Ninja Foodi and heat oil.
2. Stir in the onions and garlic. Sauté until fragrant.
3. Add the rest of the ingredients.
4. Install pressure lid. Close Ninja Foodi, press the button, choose high settings, and set time to 10 minutes.
5. Once done cooking, do a quick release.
6. Open the lid and transfer the contents into a blender. Pulse until smooth. Serve with cheese on top if desired.
7. Serve and enjoy.

- **Nutrition Info:** Calories: 103; carbohydrates:15.2 g; protein:1.9 g; fat: 3.8g

166. Tipsy Potato Chowder

Servings: 5 Servings
Cooking Time: 8 Hours
Ingredients:
- 6 cups potatoes, peeled and cubed
- 2 cups cheddar cheese, grated
- 1 ¾ cups chicken broth
- 1 can beer
- ½ cup onion, chopped
- ½ cup celery, chopped
- ½ cup carrot, chopped
- ½ cup heavy cream
- 1 clove garlic, chopped fine
- ¼ teaspoon pepper

Directions:
1. Combine all ingredients, except the cheese and cream to the cooking pot. Add lid and set to slow cooking on low. Cook 6-8 hours, stirring every so often
2. About 10 minutes before serving, coarsely mash the vegetables, leaving the soup a little chunky. Add cheese and cream and stir to combine. Cover and cook 5 minutes more or till cheese is melted. Serve.

167. Greens & Beans Soup

Servings: 8 – 10 Servings
Cooking Time: 6 Hours
Ingredients:
- 1 pound bean soup mix, rinsed and debris removed
- 6 cups chicken broth
- 6 cups mustard or collard greens, chopped
- 2 smoked turkey wings.
- 2 cups baby Portabella mushrooms
- 1 onion, chopped
- 1 can tomatoes, diced
- 1 cup carrots, cut into chunks
- 7 cloves garlic, chopped fine
- ¾ cup red wine
- 2 tablespoons Italian seasoning
- 1 teaspoon sage
- 2 bay leaves
- Salt & pepper

Directions:
1. Add all of the ingredients, but use only half the greens, to the cooking pot. Secure lid and select slow cooking on high. Cook 5 ½ hours.
2. Remove turkey wings. When cool enough to handle, remove any meat from the bones and add it back to the soup. Add remaining greens and cook another 15 minutes. Serve topped with Parmesan cheese if desired.

168. Coconut, Apple 'n Squash Chowder

Servings: 2
Cooking Time: 15 Minutes
Ingredients:
- 3/4 cup vegetable stock
- 1 cloves of garlic, minced
- 1 small carrot, diced
- 1 granny smith apple, cored and diced
- 1/2 small squash, seeded and diced
- 1/2 onion, diced
- Salt and pepper to taste
- A pinch of ground cinnamon
- 1/4 cup canned coconut milk
- A pinch of paprika powder

Directions:
1. In the Ninja Foodi, put in the vegetable stock, garlic, carrots, apples, and squash. Season with salt and pepper to taste and sprinkle with cinnamon.
2. Install pressure lid.
3. Close Ninja Foodi, press the manual button, choose high settings, and set time to 15 minutes.
4. Once done cooking, do a quick release.
5. Open the lid and press the sauté button. Stir in the coconut milk.
6. Using an immersion blender, pulse until the mixture becomes smooth.
7. Sprinkle with paprika on top.
8. Serve and enjoy.
- **Nutrition Info:**

169. Deliciously Traditional Clam Chowder

Servings: 2
Cooking Time: 17 Minutes
Ingredients:

- 2 6.5-oz cans chopped clams (reserve the clam juice)
- Water
- 2 slices bacon, chopped
- 1 1/2 tbsp butter
- 1 onion, diced
- 1 stalks celery, diced
- 1 sprig fresh thyme
- 1 cloves garlic, pressed or finely minced
- 1/2 tsp kosher salt or more
- 1/4 tsp pepper
- ½-lb potatoes, diced
- 1/2 tsp sugar
- 1/2 cup half and half
- Chopped chives, for garnish

Directions:
1. Drain the clam juice into a 2-cup measuring cup. Add enough water to make 2 cups of liquid. Set the clams and juice/water aside.
2. Press sauté button and cook bacon for 3 minutes until fat has rendered out of it, but not crispy. Add the butter, onion, celery, and thyme. Cook for 5 minutes while frequently stirring. Add the garlic, salt, and pepper. Cook for 1 minute, stirring frequently.
3. Add the potatoes, sugar (if using) and clam juice/water mixture and deglaze pot. Press stop.
4. Close Ninja Foodi, press pressure cook button, choose high settings, and set time to 4 minutes. Once done cooking, do a natural release for 3 minutes and then do a quick release. Mash the potatoes. Stir in half and half and the clams. Mix well.
5. Serve and enjoy garnished with chives.
- **Nutrition Info:** Calories: 381; carbohydrates: 32.8g; protein: 29.3g; fat: 14.7

170.Irish Lamb Stew

Servings: 6 Servings
Cooking Time: 8 Hours 15 Mins
Ingredients:
- 1 ½ pounds lamb stew meat
- 4 cups chicken broth
- 3 ½ cups cabbage, chopped
- 2 cups water
- 2 large potatoes, peeled and chopped

- 1 onion, chopped
- 1 carrot, chopped
- 1 leek, chopped
- 1 cup baby spinach
- 2 tablespoons olive oil
- 1 tablespoon fresh mint, chopped fine
- 2 sprigs rosemary
- 1 bay leaf

Directions:
1. Add 1 tablespoon of the oil to the cooking pot and set to sauté on medium heat. Sprinkle the lamb with salt and pepper and add to the pot. Cook till brown on both sides, about 8 – 10 minutes. Transfer the lamb to a plate.
2. Add the remaining oil to the pot along with the onion. Cook, stirring often, 2 minutes. Add the carrots and the leek. Cook till the vegetables start to soften, about 5 minutes.
3. Add the potatoes and the lamb to the pot. Pour in the broth and water, then add the rosemary and bay leaf. Secure the lid and select slow cooking on low. Cook 8 hours.
4. Stir in the spinach before serving. Ladle into bowls and sprinkle with mint.

171.Verde Pork Stew

Servings: 6 Servings
Cooking Time: 4 – 8 Hours
Ingredients:
- 1 – 1 ½ pound pork tenderloin
- 2 cups chicken broth
- 1 16-ounce jar salsa verde
- 1 15-ounce can black beans, rinsed and drained
- 1 teaspoon cumin

Directions:
1. Place all ingredients in the cooking pot. Set to slow cooker functions. Cook 3-4 hours on high heat, or 6-8 hours on low.
2. When pork is tender, transfer it to a bowl and shred with two forks. Return it to the pot and stir to combine. Serve garnished as desired.

172.Chili-quinoa 'n Black Bean Soup

Servings: 2
Cooking Time: 20 Minutes

Ingredients:

- 1/2 bell pepper, diced
- 1 medium-sized sweet potatoes, peeled and diced
- 1/2 onion, diced
- 1 clove garlic, minced
- 1 stalk celery, chopped
- 1 1/3 cups vegetable broth
- 1 tablespoon tomato paste
- 1/3 cup diced tomatoes
- 1/3 can black beans, rinsed and drained
- 1 teaspoon each of paprika and cumin
- Salt to taste
- 2 tbsp quinoa
- 2 cups vegetable broth

Directions:

1. Place all ingredients in the Ninja Foodi. Give a good stir.
2. Install pressure lid.
3. Close Ninja Foodi, press the pressure button, choose high settings, and set time to 20 minutes.
4. Once done cooking, do a quick release.
5. Serve and enjoy.
- **Nutrition Info:** Calories: 377; carbohydrates: 73.7g; protein: 18.1g; fat: 1.0g

173.Sweet Potato & Black Bean Stew

Servings: 6 Servings
Cooking Time: 25 Minutes
Ingredients:

- 4 cups vegetable broth
- 4 cups kale, chopped
- 3 cups sweet potatoes, peeled and cubed
- 1 can black beans, rinsed and drained
- 1 large onion, chopped
- 4 cloves garlic, chopped fine
- 3 green onions, sliced thin
- 2 radishes, sliced thin
- 2 tablespoons olive oil
- 1 tablespoon lime juice
- 2 teaspoons oregano
- 1 ½ teaspoons cumin
- 1 teaspoon garlic powder
- ½. teaspoon black pepper
- ½ teaspoon salt

- ¼ teaspoon cayenne

Directions:

1. Add the oil to the pot and set to sauté on med-high heat. Add the onions and cook till translucent, about 3 minutes. Reduce heat to medium, add the garlic and seasonings and cook for 30 seconds.
2. Add the potatoes, broth, beans and salt and bring to a low boil. Cook 15 minutes, or till potatoes are tender.
3. Turn off the heat and stir in kale, green onions and lime juice. Serve.

174.Vegan Approver Tortilla Soup

Servings: 2
Cooking Time: 40 Minutes
Ingredients:

- 1/2 cup diced onion
- 1/2 bell pepper, diced
- 1/2 jalapeno pepper, diced
- 1 1/4 cups vegetable broth
- 1/2 can tomato sauce
- 1/4 cup salsa verde
- 1/2 tablespoon tomato paste
- 1/2 can black beans, drained and rinsed
- 1/2 can pinto beans, drained and rinsed
- 1/2 cup fresh corn kernels
- ½ teaspoon chili powder
- ½ teaspoon garlic powder
- Salt and pepper to taste
- 2 tbsp heavy cream

Directions:

1. Place all ingredients in the Ninja Foodi except for the heavy cream and give a good stir.
2. Install pressure lid. Close Ninja Foodi, press the manual button, choose high settings, and set time to 20 minutes.
3. Once done cooking, do a quick release.
4. Open the lid and press the sauté button. Stir in the heavy cream and allow to simmer for 5 minutes.
5. Serve and enjoy.
- **Nutrition Info:** Calories: 341; carbohydrates: 48.7g; protein: 8.6g; fat: 12.4g

175.Lamb Provencal

Servings: 4 Servings
Cooking Time: 40 Minutes
Ingredients:

- 1 pound lamb stew meat
- 4 cups beef broth
- 2 cups mushrooms, quartered
- 2 cups sweet potatoes, peeled and cubed
- 2 cups turnips, peeled and cubed
- 1 cup dry red wine
- 1 shallot, chopped fine
- ¾ cup flour
- 2 tablespoons olive oil
- 1 tablespoon Herbes de Provence
- 2 bay leaves
- 1 sprig rosemary
- 1 teaspoon garlic, chopped fine
- ½ teaspoon salt
- a few grinds of pepper

Directions:

1. In a large bowl, mix together flour with some salt and pepper. Add the lamb and toss to coat well.
2. Add the oil to the cooking pot and set to sauté on med-high heat. When hot, add the lamb, shallot and garlic and cook till lamb begins to brown.
3. Add the broth, wine and seasonings and stir to combine. Secure the lid and set to pressure cooking on high. Set the timer for 30 minutes.
4. When the timer goes off, use quick release to remove the lid. Add the vegetables and secure the lid again. Cook on high pressure for 10 minutes.
5. Use quick release to remove the lid. Stir well and serve.

176.Seafood Stew

Servings: 4 Servings
Cooking Time: 25 Mins
Ingredients:

- 1 pound mixed lobster, shrimp and cod
- 3 ½ cups water
- 3 ½ cups tomatoes, crushed
- 2 cups potatoes, cubed
- 1 ½ cups celery, sliced
- 1 ½ cups onions, chopped
- 1 ½ cups carrots, sliced
- ¼ cups shallots, chopped
- 4 - 6 cloves of garlic, chopped fine
- 1 teaspoon salt
- 1 teaspoon pepper
- 1 teaspoon basil
- 1 teaspoon Greek seasoning
- 1 teaspoon Sriracha sauce

Directions:

1. Place all the vegetables, except the potatoes into the cooking pot. Add tomatoes, water and seasonings. Secure lid and set to pressure cooking on high. Set timer for 10 minutes.
2. When timer goes off, use quick release to remove the lid. Add the potatoes and pressure cook another 8 minutes. Use quick release again.
3. Set to sauté on medium heat. Stir in the seafood and cook till shrimp and lobster is pink and the stew is heated through, about 5 minutes. Serve.

177.Chickpea And Potato Soup

Servings: 2
Cooking Time: 15 Minutes
Ingredients:

- 1 tablespoon olive oil
- ½ onion, chopped
- 3 cloves of garlic, minced
- ½ cup chopped tomato
- 1/8 teaspoon fennel space
- ½ teaspoon onion powder
- ¼ teaspoon garlic powder
- ½ teaspoon oregano
- ¼ teaspoon cinnamon
- ½ teaspoon thyme
- 1 large potato, peeled and cubed
- ¾ cup carrots, chopped
- 1 ½ cups cooked chickpeas
- 1 cup water
- 1 cup almond milk
- 1 cup kale, chopped
- Salt and pepper to taste

Directions:

1. Press the sauté button on the Ninja Foodi and sauté the onion and garlic until fragrant.
2. Stir in the tomatoes, fennel, onion powder, garlic powder, oregano, cinnamon, and thyme. Stir until well-combined.
3. Add the rest of the ingredients. Install pressure lid. Close Ninja Foodi, press the pressure button, choose high settings, and set time to 10 minutes.
4. Once done cooking, do a quick release. Serve and enjoy.
- **Nutrition Info:** Calories: 543; carbohydrates: 91.0g; protein: 17.7g; fat: 12g

178.Shrimp & Mango Curry

Servings: 4 Servings
Cooking Time: 15 Minutes
Ingredients:
- 1 ¼ pounds shrimp, peeled and deveined
- 2 cups clam juice
- 1 can coconut milk
- 3 mangoes, chopped
- 1 onion, chopped
- 2 stalks celery, sliced
- 1 bunch scallions, sliced
- 4 cloves garlic, chopped fine
- 1 serrano chili, seeded and chopped fine
- 2 tablespoons curry powder
- 1 tablespoon olive oil
- 1 teaspoon thyme
- ¼ teaspoon salt

Directions:
1. Add oil to cooker and set to sauté on medium heat. Add onion and celery and cook, stirring often, till the onion begins to brown, about 3-5 minutes.
2. Add garlic, chili, curry powder and thyme, stir constantly and cook 30 seconds. Add the clam juice, coconut milk and mangoes and increase the heat to med-high. Bring to a simmer and cook, stirring often, for 5 minutes.
3. Add 3 cups of the soup to a blender and process till smooth. Return it to the pot and bring back to simmer. Add shrimp and cook till they turn pink, about 3 minutes. Stir in scallions and salt and serve.

179.Healthy Celery 'n Kale Soup

Servings: 2
Cooking Time: 35 Minutes
Ingredients:
- 1 teaspoon olive oil
- 1/2 onion, diced
- 1 clove garlic, minced
- 1 stalk celery, chopped
- 1 carrot, peeled and chopped
- 1 small potato, peeled and diced
- 1 teaspoon herbs de provence
- 1/2 can diced tomatoes
- 2 cups vegetable broth
- 2 cups green lentils, soaked overnight
- Salt and pepper to taste
- 1 cup kale, torn

Directions:
1. Press the sauté button on the Ninja Foodi and heat the oil.
2. Sauté the onion, garlic, and celery until fragrant.
3. Stir in the carrots, potatoes, herbs, tomatoes, vegetable broth and lentils. Season with salt and pepper to taste.
4. Install pressure lid. Close Ninja Foodi, press the pressure button, choose high settings, and set time to 30 minutes.
5. Once done cooking, do a quick release. Open the lid and stir in the kale while still hot. Serve and enjoy.
- **Nutrition Info:** Calories: 331; carbohydrates: 53g; protein: 23g; fat: 3g

180.Jamaican Chicken Stew

Servings: 6 Servings
Cooking Time: 30 Mins
Ingredients:
- Marinade
- 2 ½ – 3 pounds chicken thighs, skinless
- 1-2 green onions, chopped
- 1 teaspoon garlic, chopped fine
- ½ teaspoon ginger, grated
- ½ teaspoon white pepper
- ½ teaspoon thyme
- ½ teaspoon salt
- ½ teaspoon chicken bouillon powder
- For the stew

- 2 cups chicken broth
- 1-2 small red bell peppers, seeded and chopped
- 1 onion, chopped fine
- ¼ cup vegetable oil
- 1 tablespoon ketchup
- 2 teaspoon brown sugar
- 1 teaspoon browning sauce
- 1 teaspoon hot sauce
- 1 teaspoon smoked paprika
- ½ teaspoon thyme
- salt to taste

Directions:

1. Place chicken in a large bowl, then add all of the marinade ingredients. Mix to make sure the chicken is coated. Cover and refrigerate at least 30 minutes or overnight.
2. When ready to cook shake off any excess spice or onions from the chicken.
3. Add the oil to the cooking pot and set to sauté on medium. When the oil is hot, add the chicken and cook till chicken is browned, about 4-5 minutes. Remove the chicken to a plate and drain off excess oil.
4. Add onions, hot sauce, paprika and bell peppers to the pot. Cook, stirring often, till onion is translucent, about 2-3 minutes. Add the chicken with remaining stew ingredients and bring to a boil. Let it simmer, stirring often, till sauce thickens, about 15-20 minutes.

181.Sausage & Spinach Stew

Servings: 4 Servings
Cooking Time: 20 Minutes
Ingredients:

- 12 ounce Italian chicken sausage, fully cooked
- 4 cups chicken broth
- 1 bag spinach
- 1 can cannellini beans, rinsed and drained
- 1 cup ditalini pasta
- ½ cup dry white wine
- 4 cloves garlic, chopped
- 1 tablespoon olive oil
- Pepper
- Parmesan cheese

Directions:

1. Add oil to cooker and set to sauté on medium heat. Add the sausage and cook, stirring often, till brown, about 4-5 minutes. Remove to a plate.
2. Add the garlic and cook, stirring, 1 minute. Add the wine and simmer to deglaze the pan, about 1 minutes.
3. Add the broth and pasta and bring to a boil. Cook till pasta is tender, about 8-10 minutes. Stir in the beans, sausage and pepper and cook till heated through. Turn the cooker off and stir in the spinach. Ladle into bowls and top with Parmesan cheese before serving.

182.Venison Stew

Servings: 4 Servings
Cooking Time: 2 Hours
Ingredients:

- 1 pound venison stew meat
- 3 cups beef broth
- 4 slices bacon, cut into ½ -inch pieces
- 1 cup dry red wine
- 2 carrots, sliced
- 1 large potato, cubed
- 1 onion, chopped
- 1 stalk celery, sliced thin
- ½ cup cold water
- 3 tablespoons flour
- ½ teaspoon salt
- ¼ teaspoon thyme
- ¼ teaspoon marjoram
- ¼ teaspoon pepper

Directions:

1. Add the bacon to the pot and set cooker to sauté on med-high heat. Cook till crispy, remove to paper towel lined plate.
2. Add the venison to the pot and cook till brown on all sides. Add the broth, wine, celery, carrots and seasonings and stir to combine. Add the lid and set the cooker to slow cooking on high. Cook one hour.
3. After one hour, add the potatoes and cook till meat and vegetables are tender.
4. Stir the flour into the cold water in a small bowl, or measuring glass. Stir into the stew and continue to cook thill thickened, about 5-10 minutes. Stir in bacon just before serving.

183.Sunchoke & Asparagus Soup

Servings: 4 Servings
Cooking Time: 15 Minutes
Ingredients:
- 1 pound asparagus, cut off 1 ½ inches of the tips, discard woody ends and chop remaining into 1-inch pieces
- 3 cups vegetable broth
- ½ pound sunchokes, peeled and chopped
- 1 ½ cups potato, peeled and chopped
- 2 large shallots, peeled and sliced
- 2 tablespoons olive oil
- ½ teaspoons salt
- 1/8 teaspoon white pepper

Directions:
1. Add oil to the pot and set to sauté on medium heat. Add shallot and cook till soft. Add the vegetables along with the broth. Secure the lid and set to pressure cooking on high. Set the timer for 10 minutes. When the timer goes off, use quick release to remove the lid.
2. While the vegetables are cooking, bring a small pot of water to a boil and prepare an ice bath in a bowl. Add the asparagus tips to the boiling water and cook 2 minutes. Transfer the tips to the ice bath with a slotted spoon.
3. Once the vegetables in the cooking pot are tender, use an immersion blender to puree till smooth. Season with salt and pepper to taste.
4. To serve, ladle soup into bowls, divide the asparagus tips among them and drizzle a little olive oil over the top.

184.Spiced Potato-cauliflower Chowder

Servings: 2
Cooking Time: 7 Minutes
Ingredients:
- 1 head cauliflower, cut into florets
- 2 small red potatoes, peeled and sliced
- 4 cups vegetable stock
- 6 cloves of garlic, minced
- 1 onion, diced
- 1 cup heavy cream
- 2 bay leaves
- Salt and pepper to taste
- 2 stalks of green onions

Directions:
1. Place the cauliflower, potatoes, vegetable stock, garlic, onion, heavy cream, and bay leaves in the Ninja Foodi. Season with salt and pepper to taste.
2. Install pressure lid. Close Ninja Foodi, press the pressure button, choose high settings, and set time to 6 minutes.
3. Once done cooking, do a quick release.
4. Open the lid and stir in the green onions.
5. Serve and enjoy.
- **Nutrition Info:** Calories: 448; carbohydrates: 47.7g; protein: 10.1g; fat: 24.1g

185.Mushroom & Wild Rice Soup

Servings: 6 Servings
Cooking Time: 6 – 8 Hours
Ingredients:
- 1 pound mushrooms, halved
- 4 cups beef broth
- 2 carrots, cut into ½-inch pieces
- 1 cup frozen sweet peas, thawed
- 1 cup water
- 1 stalk celery, cut into ½-inch pieces
- ½ cup whole-grain wild rice
- 1 envelope onion soup mix
- 1 tablespoon sugar

Directions:
1. Layer mushrooms, rice, celery, carrots, soup mix and sugar in the cooking pot. Pour water and broth over top.
2. Add lid and set to slow cooking on low. Cook 5-8 hours.
3. Add the peas during the last 10 minutes of cooking. Serve.

186.White Chicken Chili

Servings: 6-8 Servings
Cooking Time: 40-50 Minutes
Ingredients:
- 4 cups chicken, cooked and chopped
- 3 ½ cups chicken broth
- 2 cans white beans, drained and rinsed
- 2 cans green chilies, diced
- 1 onion, chopped

- 2 teaspoons olive oil
- 2 teaspoons cumin
- 2 teaspoons oregano
- 1 clove garlic, chopped fine
- 1 teaspoon cayenne pepper

Directions:
1. Set cooker to sauté on med-high heat and add oil. Once oil is hot, add onion and cook 3-4 minutes or they are translucent. Add garlic and cook another minute. Add green chilies and spices and cook 2 more minutes, stirring frequently.
2. Add broth and beans. Secure lid. Set to pressure cooking function with low pressure. Set timer for 20 minutes. When timer goes off, use quick release to remove the lid.
3. Set back to sauté on low heat. Add chicken and cook 10-15 minutes, stirring occasionally. Serve garnished as desired.

187. Tuscan-style Veggie Soup

Servings: 4 Servings
Cooking Time: 20 Minutes
Ingredients:
- 3 cups vegetable broth
- 2 cups kale, chopped
- 2 cups croutons
- ½ large can tomatoes, diced
- 1 can navy beans, rinsed and drained
- 1 cup water
- 1 onion, chopped
- ½ cup fresh basil, chopped
- ½ cup Parmesan cheese
- 1 tablespoon olive oil
- 1 clove garlic, chopped fine

Directions:
1. Add oil to the pot and set cooker to sauté on medium heat. Add the onion and garlic and cook, stirring often, 3 minutes. Add the broth, water, beans and tomatoes. Bring to a boil, then reduce heat to med-low.
2. Cover and cook 10 minutes. Stir in the kale and cook 5 minutes more or till kale is tender.
3. Ladle into bowls and top with croutons and Parmesan cheese.

188. Sweet Potato 'n Garbanzo Soup

Servings: 2
Cooking Time: 10 Minutes
Ingredients:
- 1/2 yellow onion, chopped
- 1/2 tablespoon garlic, minced
- 1 can garbanzo beans, drained
- 1/2-pound sweet potatoes, peeled and chopped
- Salt and pepper to taste
- 1/2 teaspoon ground ginger
- 1/2 teaspoon ground cumin
- 1/2 teaspoon ground coriander
- 1/2 teaspoon ground cinnamon
- 2 cups vegetable broth
- 2 cups spinach, torn

Directions:
1. Place all ingredients in the Ninja Foodi except for the spinach.
2. Install pressure lid. Close Ninja Foodi, press the manual button, choose high settings, and set time to 10 minutes.
3. Once done cooking, do a quick release.
4. Open the lid and stir in the spinach. Press the sauté button and allow to simmer until the spinach wilts.
5. Serve and enjoy.
- **Nutrition Info:** Calories: 165; carbohydrates: 32.3g; protein: 6.3g; fat: 1.1g

189. Beefy White Cream Soup

Servings: 2
Cooking Time: 17 Minutes
Ingredients:
- ½ pounds stew meat
- 2 cups beef broth
- 1 1/2 tablespoons Worcestershire sauce
- ½ teaspoon Italian seasoning
- 1 teaspoon onion powder
- 1 teaspoons garlic powder
- 1/4 cup sour cream
- 3 ounces mushrooms, sliced
- Salt and pepper to taste
- 2 ounces short noodles, blanched

Directions:
1. Place the meat, broth, Worcestershire sauce, Italian seasoning, onion powder, garlic

powder, sour cream, and mushrooms. Season with salt and pepper to taste.

2. Install pressure lid. Close Ninja Foodi, press the pressure button, choose high settings, and set time to 12 minutes.
3. Once done cooking, do a quick release. Open the lid and press the sauté button. Stir in the noodles and allow to simmer for 5 minutes.
4. Serve and enjoy.

- **Nutrition Info:** Calories: 599 ; carbohydrates: 65g; protein: 39.6g; fat: 20.1g

190.Cheesy Onion Soup

Servings: 4 Servings
Cooking Time: 10 Minutes
Ingredients:
- 2 ¼ cups sharp cheddar cheese, grated
- 1 Vidalia onion, sliced thin
- 1 can chicken broth
- 1 cup milk
- ¼ cup celery, chopped fine
- ¼ cup dry white wine
- 2 tablespoons butter
- 2 tablespoons flour
- 1 tablespoon chives, chopped
- ½ teaspoon pepper
- ½ teaspoon dry mustard

Directions:
1. Add butter to the cooking pot and set to sauté on medium heat. Once melted, add onion and celery and cook 3 minutes, stirring often.
2. Stir in flour, pepper and mustard. Slowly stir in the milk, broth and wine. Bring to a boil and cook, stirring, one minute.
3. Stir in the cheese, reduce heat to low and while stirring constantly, cook till cheese is melted. Ladle into bowls and garnish with chopped chives.

DESSERT RECIPES

191. Coconut Cake

Servings: 6 Servings
Cooking Time: 25 Minutes
Ingredients:

- 8 Tbsp butter
- ½ cup Baking Stevia
- 1 egg
- 1 tsp vanilla
- 1 cup coconut flour
- ½ cup almond flour
- ½ cup shredded coconut, unsweetened
- 2 tsp baking powder
- 1 tsp salt
- 1 cup chopped strawberries
- ½ cup buttermilk

Directions:

1. Use an electric mixer to cream the butter and stevia together until they are light and fluffy.
2. Mix the vanilla and eggs in a small bowl then add to the mixer with the butter blend until just combined
3. Add the remaining dry ingredients to the mixer and fold together by hand. Add the buttermilk and mix until smooth.
4. Pour the cake batter into your Ninja Foodi and place the lid on.
5. Press the air crisp button and set the temperature to 350 degrees and program the timer to 25 minutes.
6. Once cooked, a toothpick should come out of the center of the cake cleanly. Allow to cool and serve.
- **Nutrition Info:** Calories: 197 g, Carbohydrates: 6g , Protein: 3g, Fat: 18 g, Sugar: 2g, Sodium: 559 mg

192. Fruity And Tasty Vegan Crumble

Servings: 2
Cooking Time: 15 Minutes
Ingredients:

- 1 medium apple, finely diced
- ½ cup frozen blueberries, strawberries, or peaches
- ¼ cup plus 1 tablespoon sear button rice flour

- 2 tablespoons sugar
- ½ teaspoon ground cinnamon
- 2 tablespoons nondairy butter

Directions:

1. Lightly grease pot of Ninja Foodi with cooking spray.
2. Spread frozen blueberries and apple slices on bottom of pot.
3. In a bowl, whisk well butter, cinnamon, sugar, and flour. Sprinkle over fruit. If needed, sprinkle extra flour to cover exposed fruit.
4. For 15 minutes, bake at 350 ºF
5. Serve and enjoy.
- **Nutrition Info:** Calories: 281; carbs: 40.1g; protein: 2.0g; fat: 12.5g

193. Pineapple Pecan Bread Pudding

Servings: Serves 4
Cooking Time: 30 – 35 Minutes
Ingredients:

- 2 cups French bread, cubed
- 14 ounce can crushed pineapple, drained
- 1 cup sugar
- ½ cup butter, soft
- 4 eggs
- ¼ cup pecans, chopped
- ½ teaspoon cinnamon

Directions:

1. Butter a 1 ½ quart baking dish that fits inside the cooking pot. Add the rack to the bottom of the pot.
2. In a large bowl, on medium speed, beat butter sugar and cinnamon for 1 minutes, scraping sides of the bowl frequently. Add eggs and beat 2 minutes, or till light and fluffy. Fold in remaining ingredients and pour into prepared baking dish.
3. Place the dish on the rack and add the Tender Crisp lid. Set the temperature to 330 degrees and bake 30-35 minutes, or it passes the toothpick test. Serve warm dusted with powdered sugar.

194. Balsamic Roasted Strawberries

Servings: 4 Servings
Cooking Time: 10 Minutes

Ingredients:

- 4 Cups whole Strawberries
- ½ cup balsamic vinegar
- 2 Tbsp stevia

Directions:

1. Place all the ingredients into the pot of the Ninja Foodi and close the crisper lid.
2. Press the air crisp button and set the temperature to 350 degrees and program the timer to 10 minutes.
3. Serve hot or chilled
- **Nutrition Info:** Calories: 172g, Carbohydrates: 21g, Protein: 0g, Fat: 0g, Sugar: 37g, Sodium: 20mg

195.Surprising Campfire S'mores

Servings: 4
Cooking Time: 14 Minutes
Ingredients:

- 4 Graham Crackers
- 4 marshmallows
- 2 (1½ oz. each) chocolate bars

Directions:

1. Place Cook and Crisp basket in the pot, close crisping lid
2. Pre-heat your pot by setting it to 350 degrees F on Air Crisp mode, for 5 minutes
3. Break graham crackers into half and place half of the chocolate bar on one half of Graham Cracker
4. Add marshmallow and top with remaining graham cracker half
5. Repeat with remaining ingredients to create the S'Mores
6. Use aluminum foil to wrap each S'More individually, place all 4 foil-wrapped S'Mores in your pre-heated Cook and Crisp Basket
7. Place Crisping Lid and select the Air Crisp mode, cook for 4 minutes at 350 degrees F
8. Carefully unwrap the S'mores, serve and enjoy!
- **Nutrition Info:** 152 Calories, 7g fat, 24g carbs, 1g protein

196.Crunchy Cinnamon Topped Peaches

Servings: 2
Cooking Time: 30 Minutes

Ingredients:

- 2 cups sliced peaches, frozen
- 1 1/2 tablespoons sugar
- 1 tablespoon flour, white
- 1/2 teaspoon sugar, white
- 2 tbsp flour, white
- 3 tbsp oats, dry rolled
- 1 1/2 tablespoons butter, unsalted
- 1/2 teaspoons cinnamon
- 1 ½ tablespoons pecans, chopped

Directions:

1. Lightly grease the pot of Ninja Foodi with cooking spray. Mix in a tsp cinnamon, 2 tbsp flour, 3 tbsp sugar, and peaches.
2. For 20 minutes, bake on 300 ºF.
3. Mix the rest of the ingredients: in a bowl. Pour over peaches.
4. Bake for 10 minutes more at 330 ºF.
5. Serve and enjoy.
- **Nutrition Info:** Calories: 435; carbs: 74.1g; protein: 4.3g; fat: 13.4g

197.Raspberry Mug Cake

Servings: 2 Servings
Cooking Time: 10 Minutes
Ingredients:

- 2/3 cup almond flour
- 2 eggs
- 2 Tbsp maple syrup
- 1 tsp vanilla
- 1/8 tsp salt
- 1 cup fresh raspberries

Directions:

1. Mix all the ingredients together except the raspberries. Fold well to ensure no lumps.
2. Fold in raspberries
3. Pour the batter into two 8 oz mason jars and cover the jars with foil.
4. Place the metal trivet into the Ninja Foodi and add 1 cup of water to the bowl.
5. Place the two mason jars on top of the trivet and close the pressure cooker top. Seal the steamer valve and set the timer to 10 minutes
6. Let the pressure naturally release and then open the lid and enjoy the warm cake.

- **Nutrition Info:** Calories: 215g, Carbohydrates: 10g, Protein: 9g, Fat: 10g, Sugar: 16g, Sodium: 82mg

198.Noodle Kugel

Servings: 10 Servings
Cooking Time: 6 Hours
Ingredients:
- 1 pound egg noodles, uncooked
- 1 bag frozen peaches, thawed and chopped
- 1 can coconut milk
- 1 cup sugar
- 3 eggs
- ¼ cup raisins
- 3 tablespoons orange liquor
- 2 teaspoons cinnamon

Directions:
1. Soak raisins in the liquor in a small bowl for 20 minutes.
2. Lightly spray the pot with cooking spray. Add milk, sugar, 1 teaspoon cinnamon and eggs to the pot and stir to combine.
3. Add the noodles, raisins with liquor and peaches to the egg mixture and stir to combine. Sprinkle the remaining teaspoon of cinnamon on the top. Add the lid and set slow cooking on low heat. Cook 6 hours.

199.Coconutty-blueberry Cake

Servings: 2
Cooking Time: 10 Minutes
Ingredients:
- 1/4 cup coconut flour
- 2 large eggs
- 1/2 teaspoon baking soda
- 1/4 cup coconut milk
- 1/4 teaspoon lemon zest

Directions:
1. Combine all ingredients in a mixing bowl.
2. Pour into two mugs. Cover top of mugs securely with foil.
3. Place a steam rack in the Ninja Foodi and pour a cup of water.
4. Place the mug on the steam rack.
5. Install pressure lid. Close the lid, press the steam button, and adjust the time to 10 minutes.
6. Do a natural pressure release.

- **Nutrition Info:** Calories: 259; carbohydrates: 10.3g; protein: 7.2g; fat: 20.9g

200.Sweet Sticky Coco-rice

Servings: 2
Cooking Time: 20 Minutes
Ingredients:
- 1/2 cup Thai sweet rice
- ¾ cup water
- 1/2 can full fat coconut milk
- A pinch of salt
- 2 tablespoons pure sugar
- 1/4 teaspoon cornstarch + 1 tablespoon water
- 1 small mango, sliced
- Sesame seeds for garnish

Directions:
1. Place rice and water in the Ninja Foodi.
2. Install pressure lid. Close the lid and press the pressure button. Cook on high for 5 minutes.
3. Turn off the Ninja Foodi and do natural pressure release for 10 minutes.
4. While the rice is cooking, place the coconut milk, salt, and sugar in a saucepan. Heat over medium heat for 10 minutes while stirring constantly.
5. Once the Ninja Foodi lid can be open, add the coconut milk mixture. Stir well. Place a clean kitchen towel over the opening of the lid and let it rest for 10 minutes.
6. Meanwhile, mix cornstarch with water and add to the rice. Press the sauté button and mix until the rice becomes creamy and thick.
7. Serve with mango slices and sesame seeds.

- **Nutrition Info:** Calories: 318; carbohydrates: 36.5g; protein: 3.5g; fat: 17.5g

201.Hot Fudge Cake

Servings: 6 Servings
Cooking Time: 2 – 2 ½ Hours
Ingredients:
- 1 ½ cups hot water
- 1cup flour
- ¾ cup brown sugar, packed
- ½ cup sugar

- ½ cup milk
- ½ cup nuts, chopped
- ¼ cup baking cocoa
- 2 tablespoons baking cocoa
- 2 tablespoons vegetable oil
- 2 teaspoons baking powder
- 1 teaspoon vanilla
- ½ teaspoon salt

Directions:
1. Lightly spray the pot with cooking spray.
2. In a medium bowl mix flour, sugar, 2 tablespoons cocoa, baking powder and salt together. Stir in milk, oil and vanilla till smooth. Stir in nuts and spread the batter evenly in the cooking pot.
3. In a small bowl, whisk together brown sugar, ¼ cup cocoa and hot water till smooth. Pour over batter in the cooking pot.
4. Add the lid and select slow cooking on high. Cook the cake 2 – 21/2 hours or it passes the toothpick test.
5. Turn off the cooker and let the cake rest, uncovered 30-40 minutes. Serve.

202.Caramel Apple Chimichangas

Servings: 1 Dozen
Cooking Time: 6 Mins
Ingredients:
- 12 10-inch flour tortillas
- 7 Granny Smith apples, peeled, cored and sliced
- 1 lemon, juice and zest
- ¾ cup light brown sugar
- ¼ cup flour
- ¾ teaspoon ground cinnamon
- Cinnamon sugar
- Caramel sauce

Directions:
1. Preheat air fryer to 400 degrees.
2. Mix the brown sugar, flour and cinnamon together in small bowl.
3. In a large bowl, toss the apples with the lemon juice, then stir in the sugar mixture making sure to coat all of the apples.
4. Warm the tortillas so they are soft enough to fold. Place ½ - ¾ cup apples in the center of tortilla and fold like a burrito. You can seal the edge with water or use toothpicks.

5. Lightly spray the outsides with cooking spray and sprinkle with the cinnamon sugar.
6. Cook them in batches in the fryer, 6-7 minutes, turning halfway through.
7. Drizzle with the caramel sauce, or serve them with the caramel sauce for dipping.

203.Bananas Foster

Servings: 6 – 8 Servings
Cooking Time: 2 Hours
Ingredients:
- 7 bananas, not too ripe, sliced into ½-inch pieces
- 6 tablespoons honey
- Juice of 1 lemon
- 2 tablespoons coconut oil, melted
- 1 teaspoon rum extract
- ½ teaspoon cinnamon
- 1 tablespoon coconut oil, melted (unrefined coconut oil)
- 3 tablespoon honey
- Juice from 1/2 lemon
- 1/4 teaspoon cinnamon
- 5 bananas, medium firmness, 1/2" slices
- 1/2 teaspoon 100% Rum Extract (optional)

Directions:
1. Add the coconut oil, honey, lemon juice and cinnamon to the cooking pot. Stir to combine. Add bananas and toss gently to coat. Add the lid and set to slow cooking on low. Cook 1 ½ - 2 hours.
2. Just before serving, add the rum extract. Serve over vanilla ice cream, or topped with whip cream.

204.Lemon Mousse

Servings: 2
Cooking Time: 22 Minutes
Ingredients:
- 1 oz. softened cream cheese
- ½ c. heavy cream
- 1/8 c. fresh lemon juice
- ½ tsp. lemon liquid stevia
- 2 pinches salt

Directions:
1. Mix together cream cheese, heavy cream, lemon juice, salt and stevia in a bowl.

2. Pour into the ramekins and transfer the ramekins in the pot of Ninja Foodi.
3. Press "Bake/Roast" and bake for about 12 minutes at 350 degrees F.
4. Pour into the serving glasses and refrigerate for at least 3 hours before serving.
- **Nutrition Info:** 305 calories, 31g fat, 2.7g carbs, 5g protein

205.Nut Porridge

Servings: 4
Cooking Time: 20 Minutes
Ingredients:
- 4 tsps. melted coconut oil
- 1 c. halved pecans
- 2 c. water
- 2 tbsps. stevia
- 1 c. raw cashew nuts, unsalted

Directions:
1. Put the cashew nuts and pecans in the food processor and pulse until chunked.
2. Put the nuts mixture into the pot and stir in water, coconut oil and stevia.
3. Press "Sauté" on Ninja Foodi and cook for about 15 minutes.
4. Dish out and serve immediately.
- **Nutrition Info:** 260 calories, 22.9g fat, 12.7g carbs, 5.6g protein

206.Nutty Cinnamon 'n Cranberry Cake

Servings: 2
Cooking Time: 25 Minutes
Ingredients:
- 2 tbsp cashew milk (or use any dairy or non-dairy milk you prefer)
- 1 medium egg
- 1/2 tsp vanilla extract
- 1/2 cup almond flour
- 2 tbsp monk fruit (or use your preferred sweetener)
- 1/4 tsp baking powder
- 1/4 tsp cinnamon
- 1/8 tsp salt
- 3 tbsp fresh cranberries
- 2 tbsp cup chopped pecans

Directions:
1. In blender, add all wet ingredients: and mix well. Add all dry ingredients: except for

cranberries and pecans. Blend well until smooth.
2. Lightly grease baking pot of Ninja Foodi with cooking spray. Pour in batter. Drizzle cranberries on top and then followed by pecans.
3. For 20 minutes, cook on 330 ºF.
4. Let stand for 5 minutes.
5. Serve and enjoy.
- **Nutrition Info:** Calories: 98; carbs: 11.7g; protein: 1.7g; fat: 4.9g

207.Almond Cake

Servings: 8 Servings
Cooking Time: 25 Minutes
Ingredients:
- 8 Tbsp butter
- ½ cup Baking Stevia
- 1 egg
- 1 tsp vanilla
- 2 cups almond flour
- 2 tsp baking powder
- 1 tsp salt
- 1 cup chopped Almonds
- ½ cup buttermilk

Directions:
1. Use an electric mixer to cream the butter and stevia together until they are light and fluffy.
2. Mix the vanilla and eggs in a small bowl then add to the mixer with the butter blend until just combined
3. Add the remaining dry ingredients to the mixer and fold together by hand. Add the buttermilk and mix until smooth.
4. Add the almonds to the batter and mix briefly.
5. Pour the cake batter into your Ninja Foodi and place the lid on.
6. Press the air crisp button and set the temperature to 350 degrees and program the timer to 25 minutes.
7. Once cooked, a toothpick should come out of the center of the cake cleanly. Allow to cool and serve.
- **Nutrition Info:** Calories: 295 g, Carbohydrates: 6g , Protein: 7g, Fat: 29 g, Sugar: 1g, Sodium: 165 mg

208.Carrot Pecan

Servings: 6 Servings
Cooking Time: 25 Minutes
Ingredients:

- 8 Tbsp butter
- ½ cup Baking Stevia
- 1 egg
- 1 tsp vanilla
- 1 cup almond flour
- 1 cup pecan flour
- 1 cup shredded carrots
- 2 tsp baking powder
- 1 tsp salt
- ¼ cup buttermilk

Directions:

1. Use an electric mixer to cream the butter and stevia together until they are light and fluffy.
2. Mix the vanilla and eggs in a small bowl then add to the mixer with the butter blend until just combined
3. Add the remaining dry ingredients to the mixer and fold together by hand. Add the buttermilk and mix until smooth.
4. Pour the cake batter into your Ninja Foodi and place the lid on.
5. Press the air crisp button and set the temperature to 350 degrees and program the timer to 25 minutes.
6. Once cooked, a toothpick should come out of the center of the cake cleanly. Allow to cool and serve.

- **Nutrition Info:** Calories: 334 g, Carbohydrates: 17g, Protein: 5g, Fat: 29 g, Sugar: 5g, Sodium: 722 mg

209.Turtle Fudge Pudding

Servings: 6 Servings
Cooking Time: 2 ½ - 3 Hours
Ingredients:

- 1 2/3 cups hot water
- 1 ½ cups Bisquick
- 1 cup sugar
- ¾ cup caramel topping
- ½ cup unsweetened baking cocoa
- ½ cup milk
- ½ cup pecans, chopped

Directions:

1. Place rack in the bottom of the cooking pot. Lightly spray a deep baking dish that will fit inside the cooker.
2. In a large bowl, mix Bisquick, ½ cup sugar and the cocoa till combined. Stir in milk and ½ the caramel till well blended. Pour into prepared baking dish and lower on to the rack.
3. Pour the hot water over the top of the chocolate mixture and sprinkle with the remaining ½ cup sugar.
4. Add the lid and set to slow cooking on low. Cook 2 ½ - 3 hours or the top springs back when lightly touched. Turn off the cooker and let stand, uncovered 20 minutes. Serve warm drizzled with remaining caramel and sprinkle with pecans.

210.Chocolate Peanut Butter Cups

Servings: 3
Cooking Time: 40 Minutes
Ingredients:

- 1 c. butter
- ¼ c. heavy cream
- 2 oz. chocolate, unsweetened
- ¼ c. peanut butter, separated
- 4 packets stevia

Directions:

1. Melt the peanut butter and butter in a bowl and stir in unsweetened chocolate, stevia and heavy cream.
2. Mix thoroughly and pour the mixture in a baking mold.
3. Put the baking mold in the Ninja Foodi and press "Bake/Roast".
4. Set the timer for about 30 minutes at 360 degrees F and dish out to serve.

- **Nutrition Info:** 479 calories, 51.5g fat, 7.7g carbs, 5.2g protein

211.Reece's Cookie Bars

Servings: 8-10 Bars
Cooking Time: 1-2 Hours
Ingredients:

- 1 1/3 cup graham cracker crumbs
- 1 cup chocolate chips
- 1 cup peanut butter chips

- 1 can sweetened condensed milk
- ½ cup butter, melted

Directions:

1. In a small bowl, mix together cracker crumbs and butter.
2. Spray cooker with cooking spray. Press cracker mixture on the bottom. Pour milk over crust then sprinkle both chips over the milk.
3. Add lid and select slow cooking on high. Set timer for 1 hour. Bars are done with edges are golden brown. Let cool then cut into bars.

212.Cream Crepes

Servings: 6
Cooking Time: 26 Minutes
Ingredients:

- 1½ tsps. Splenda
- 3 organic eggs
- 3 tbsps. coconut flour
- ½ cup heavy cream
- 3 tbsps. melted coconut oil, divided

Directions:

1. Mix together 1½ tablespoons of coconut oil, Splenda, eggs and salt in a bowl and beat until well combined.
2. Add the coconut flour slowly and continuously beat.
3. Stir in the heavy cream and beat continuously until well combined.
4. Press "Sauté" on Ninja Foodi and pour about ¼ of the mixture in the pot.
5. Sauté for about 2 minutes on each side and dish out.
6. Repeat with the remaining mixture in batches and serve.
- **Nutrition Info:** 145 calories, 13.1g fat, 4g carbs, 3.5g protein

213.Excellent Strawberry Toast Pastries

Servings: 8
Cooking Time: 30 Minutes
Ingredients:

- 1 refrigerated pie crust, at room temperature
- ¼ c. simple strawberry jam
- Vanilla icing

- Rainbow sprinkles

Directions:

1. Place Cook and Crisp basket in the pot and close the crisping lead, pre-heat at 350 degrees F on Air Crisp mode for 5 minutes
2. Roll out pie crust on a lightly floured surface, shaping it into a large rectangle, cut dough into 8 rectangles
3. Spoon a tablespoon of jam to the center of each of 4 dough rectangles, leaving ½ inch border
4. Brush edges of filled dough with water, top each with the other 4 dough rectangles and gently press edges to seal
5. Place pastries in your pre-heated basket and coat with cooking spray
6. Arrange pastries in the Cook and Crisp basket in a single layer
7. Close crisping lid and Air Crisp for 10 minutes at 350 degrees F
8. Repeat until all pastries are done, frost pastries with vanilla icing and top with sprinkles
9. Enjoy!
- **Nutrition Info:** 363 calories, 15g fat, 55g carbs, 2g protein

214.Cherry Cobbler

Servings: 10 – 12 Servings
Cooking Time: 5 – 8 Hours
Ingredients:

- 1 box yellow cake mix
- 2 cans cherry pie filling
- ½ cup butter, melted
- ½ cup almonds, sliced and toasted
- 1 tablespoon water

Directions:

1. Lightly spray the cooking pot with cooking spray.
2. Dump the pie filling into the pot. Sprinkle the cake mix over the cherries then add the almonds.
3. Drizzle the melted butter over the top. Using knife, cut through the ingredients to marble them do not mix. Sprinkle water over the top.
4. Place 2-3 paper towels over the cooker then add the lid. Set to slow cooking. The cobbler

will be done in 3-5 hours on high, or 5-8 hours on low. Cobbler is done with the cake parts are set but not sticky. Serve warm.

215.Fudge Divine

Servings: 24
Cooking Time: 6 Hours 20 Minutes
Ingredients:
- ½ tsp. organic vanilla extract
- 1 c. heavy whipping cream
- 2 oz. softened butter
- 2 oz. chopped 70% dark chocolate

Directions:
1. Press "Sauté" and "Md:Hi" on Ninja Foodi and add vanilla and heavy cream.
2. Sauté for about 5 minutes and select "Lo".
3. Sauté for about 10 minutes and add butter and chocolate.
4. Sauté for about 2 minutes and transfer this mixture in a serving dish.
5. Refrigerate it for few hours and serve chilled.
- **Nutrition Info:** 292 calories, 26.2g fat, 8.2g carbs, 5.2g protein

216.Easy Peasy Applesauce

Servings: 2
Cooking Time: 8 Minutes
Ingredients:
- 2 medium apples, peeled and cored
- 1 cup water
- 2 teaspoons cinnamon, ground

Directions:
1. Place the apples in the Ninja Foodi. Pour in the water.
2. Install pressure lid. Close the lid and press the manual button. Cook on high for 8 minutes.
3. Do natural pressure release and open the lid.
4. Remove the excess water. Place the apples in a blender and process until smooth.
5. Add the rest of the ingredients.
6. Serve chilled.
- **Nutrition Info:** Calories: 108; carbohydrates: 25.7g; protein: 0.5g; fat: 0.3g

217.Flourless Chocolate Brownies

Servings: 4
Cooking Time: 42 Minutes
Ingredients:
- 3 eggs
- ½ c. butter
- ½ c. chocolate chips, sugar-free
- 2 scoops stevia
- 1 tsp. vanilla extract

Directions:
1. Whisk together eggs, stevia and vanilla extract.
2. Transfer this mixture in the blender and blend until frothy.
3. Put the butter and chocolate in the pot of Ninja Foodi and press "Sauté".
4. Sauté for about 2 minutes until the chocolate is melted.
5. Add the melted chocolate mixture to the egg mixture.
6. Pour the mixture in the baking mold and transfer the baking mold in the Ninja Foodi.
7. Press "Bake/Roast" and set the timer for about 30 minutes at 360 degrees F.
8. Bake for about 30 minutes and dish out.
9. Cut into equal square pieces and serve with whipped cream.
- **Nutrition Info:** 266 calories, 26.9g fat, 2.5g carbs, 4.5g protein

218.Vanilla Yogurt

Servings: 2
Cooking Time: 3 Hours 20 Minutes
Ingredients:
- ½ c. full-fat milk
- ¼ c. yogurt starter
- 1 c. heavy cream
- ½ tbsp. pure vanilla extract
- 2 scoops stevia

Directions:
1. Pour milk in the pot of Ninja Foodi and stir in heavy cream, vanilla extract and stevia.
2. Allow the yogurt to sit and press "Slow Cooker" and cook on Low for about 3 hours.
3. Add the yogurt starter in 1 cup of milk and return this mixture to the pot.
4. Lock the lid and wrap the Ninja Foodi in two small towels.

5. Let sit for about 9 hours and allow the yogurt to culture.
6. Dish out in a serving bowl or refrigerate to serve.
- **Nutrition Info:** 292 calories, 26.2g fat, 8.2g carbs, 5.2g protein

219.Key Lime Curd

Servings: 6 Servings
Cooking Time: 10 Minutes
Ingredients:
- 3 oz butter
- ½ cup baking stevia
- 2 eggs
- 2 egg yolks
- 2/3 cup key lime juice
- 2 tsp lime zest

Directions:
1. Blend the butter and stevia then add in the eggs slowly, creating an emulsion.
2. Add the key lime juice and zest and the separate into mason jars
3. Add 1 ½ cups of water to the bottom of the Ninja Foodi and place the mason jars on top of the metal trivet inside the pot.
4. Place the pressure cooker lid on the pot and set the pressure cooker function to high pressure for 10 minutes. Let the pressure release naturally after the cooking time is completed.
5. Let cool and then enjoy.
- **Nutrition Info:** Calories: 151g, Carbohydrates: 3g, Protein: 3g, Fat: 15g, Sugar: 1g, Sodium: 109mg

220.Almond Cheese Cake

Servings: 6 Servings
Cooking Time: 20 Minutes
Ingredients:
- Crust: ½ cup almond flour
- 2 Tbsp stevia
- 2 Tbsp melted butter
- Filling: 16 oz cream cheese
- ½ cup baking stevia
- 1 egg
- 2 egg yolks
- ¼ cup sour cream
- ¾ cup heavy cream

- 1 tsp almond extract

Directions:
1. In a small bowl, mix all the ingredients for the crust together. Press the crust into a 7" spring form pan wrapped in foil. Set aside
2. Add the cream cheese, stevia and cocoa powder to a food processor and blend. Add the egg and yolks and blend again. Add remaining ingredients and mix just to combine. Pour cheesecake mix on top of the prepared crust.
3. Place the pan in the Ninja Foodi bowl on top of the metal trivet. Add 2 cups of water to the bowl under the cake. Place the pressure cooker lid on and set it to high pressure for 20 minutes. Allow the pot to naturally release the pressure once he cooking time is done. Chill and then serve.
- **Nutrition Info:** Calories: 474g, Carbohydrates: 10g, Protein:8g, Fat: 46g, Sugar: 4g, Sodium: 338g

221.Blueberry & Peach Streusel Pie

Servings: 6-8 Servings
Cooking Time: 20 - 35 Minutes
Ingredients:
- 1 pie crust
- 3 peaches, peeled and sliced
- 1 ½ cups fresh blueberries, rinsed & dried
- 2-3 tablespoons tapioca, quick cooking
- 1 ½ tablespoons honey
- 1 tablespoon lemon zest
- 1 tablespoon lemon juice
- 1 egg white, lightly beaten
- 1 ½ teaspoons vanilla
- 1 teaspoon cinnamon
- Streusel Topping:
- ½ cup butter, cubed
- ½ cup quick cooking oats
- ½ cup sugar
- ¼ cup flour
- ¼ cup almonds, chopped

Directions:
1. Preheat air fryer to 340 degrees. Lightly oil a ceramic pie plate that fits inside the cooker.
2. Add the fruit, spices, zest, juice and tapioca to a large bowl and stir well.

3. Add the topping ingredients to a bowl and mix with a fork, or pastry cutter, till it comes together.

4. Roll the pie crust out, or if store bought, unfold it into the prepared pan. Brush the entire crust with the egg white. Add the fruit mixture and spread evenly.

5. Sprinkle the topping over the fruit. Add the rack to the cooking pot and place the pie on it. Bake 20-35 minutes and the crust is cooked. Cool and serve.

222.Lemon Ricotta Cake

Servings: 6 Servings
Cooking Time: 20 Minutes
Ingredients:
- Crust: ¼ cup almond flour
- ¼ cup coconut flour
- 2 Tbsp stevia
- 2 Tbsp melted butter
- Filling: 8 oz cream cheese
- ½ cup baking stevia
- 8 ounces ricotta
- 1 egg and 2 egg yolks
- ¼ cup sour cream
- ¾ cup heavy cream
- 2 Tsp lemon zest
- 1 tsp vanilla

Directions:
1. In a small bowl, mix all the ingredients for the crust together. Press the crust into a 7" spring form pan wrapped in foil. Set aside

2. Add the cream cheese, stevia and ricotta to a food processor and blend. Add the egg and yolks and blend again. Add remaining ingredients and mix just to combine. Pour cheesecake mix on top of the prepared crust.

3. Place the pan in the Ninja Foodi bowl on top of the metal trivet. Add 2 cups of water to the bowl under the cake. Place the pressure cooker lid on and set it to high pressure for 20 minutes. Allow the pot to naturally release the pressure once he cooking time is done. Chill and then serve.

- **Nutrition Info:** Calories: 483 g, Carbohydrates: 10g , Protein: 7g, Fat: 36 g, Sugar: 4g, Sodium: 338g

223.Crème Brûlée

Servings: 4
Cooking Time: 25 Minutes
Ingredients:
- 1 c. heavy cream
- ½ tbsp. vanilla extract
- 3 egg yolks
- 1 pinch salt
- ¼ c. stevia

Directions:
1. Mix together egg yolks, vanilla extract, heavy cream and salt in a bowl and beat until combined.

2. Divide the mixture into 4 greased ramekins evenly and transfer the ramekins in the basket of Ninja Foodi.

3. Press "Bake/Roast" and set the timer for about 15 minutes at 365 degrees F.

4. Remove from the Ninja Foodi and cover the ramekins with a plastic wrap.

5. Refrigerate to chill for about 3 hours and serve chilled.

- **Nutrition Info:** 149 calories, 14.5g fat, 1.6g carbs, 2.6g protein

224.Strawberry Cake

Servings: 6 Servings
Cooking Time: 25 Minutes
Ingredients:
- 8 Tbsp butter
- ½ cup Baking Stevia
- 1 egg
- 1 tsp vanilla
- 2 cups almond flour
- 2 tsp baking powder
- 1 tsp salt
- 1 cup chopped strawberries
- ½ cup buttermilk

Directions:
1. Use an electric mixer to cream the butter and stevia together until they are light and fluffy.

2. Mix the vanilla and eggs in a small bowl then add to the mixer with the butter blend. Ix until just combined

3. In a separate bowl, toss the raspberries and ¼ cup almond flour to coat the berries.

4. Add the remaining dry ingredients to the mixer and fold together by hand. Add the buttermilk and mix until smooth.
5. Add the Strawberries to the batter and mix briefly.
6. Pour the cake batter into your Ninja Foodi and place the lid on.
7. Press the air crisp button and set the temperature to 350 degrees and program the timer to 25 minutes.
8. Once cooked, a toothpick should come out of the center of the cake cleanly. Allow to cool and serve.
- **Nutrition Info:** Calories: 216g, Carbohydrates: 3g , Protein: 4g, Fat: 21g, Sugar: 3g, Sodium: 538 g

225.Lemon Sponge Pie

Servings: 8 Servings
Cooking Time: 35 – 40 Minutes
Ingredients:
- 1 pie crust
- 1 ½ cups sugar
- 1 cup milk
- 2/3 cups lemon juice
- 1/3 cup flour
- 3 eggs, separated
- ¼ teaspoon salt

Directions:
1. Place the rack in the bottom of the cooking pot. Unfold the pie crust into a pie pan that fits inside the pot.
2. In a large mixing bowl, beat egg whites till stiff peaks form, set aside.
3. In a separate mixing bowl, beat yolks, lemon juice and milk till combined. Add sugar, flour and salt and beat till smooth.
4. Fold lemon mixture into egg whites, until thoroughly blended. Pour into pie crust. Carefully lower the dish onto the rack in the pot. Add the Tender Crisp lid and set temperature to 330 degrees. Bake 35-40 minutes, or till golden brown.
5. Carefully remove the pie from the pot and cool completely. Cover loosely and refrigerate till the filling sets. Serve.

226.Chocolate Mug Cake

Servings: 2 Servings
Cooking Time: 10 Minutes
Ingredients:
- 2/3 cup almond flour
- ¼ cup cocoa powder
- 2 eggs
- 2 Tbsp maple syrup
- 1 tsp vanilla
- ¼ tsp salt

Directions:
1. Mix all the ingredients together. Fold well to ensure no lumps.
2. Pour the batter into two 8 oz mason jars and cover the jars with foil.
3. Place the metal trivet into the Ninja Foodi and add 1 cup of water to the bowl.
4. Place the two mason jars on top of the trivet and close the pressure cooker top. Seal the steamer valve and set the timer to 10 minutes
5. Let the pressure naturally release and then open the lid and enjoy the warm cake.
- **Nutrition Info:** Calories: 208g, Carbohydrates: 22g, Protein: 10g, Fat: 11g, Sugar: 16g, Sodium: 1238mg

227.Banana Bundt Cake

Servings: 4 -6 Servings
Cooking Time: 30 Minutes
Ingredients:
- 1 cup flour
- 1 ripe banana, mashed
- 1/3 cup brown sugar, packed
- ¼ cup butter, soft
- 1 egg
- 2-3 tablespoons walnuts, chopped
- 2 tablespoons honey
- ½ teaspoon cinnamon
- Pinch of salt

Directions:
1. Preheat air fryer to 320 degrees. Lightly spray a small ring cake pan with cooking spray.
2. Place the butter and sugar in a mixing bowl and beat till creamy. Add egg, banana and honey and stir till smooth.

3. Add the dry ingredients and stir to mix well. Pour into prepared pan.
4. Add the rack to the bottom of the cooking pot and place pan on it. Add the Tender Crisp lid and bake 30 minutes or it passes the toothpick test.
5. Carefully remove the pan from the cooker and let cool 10 minutes before transferring to a serving plate. Garnish if desired.

228.Blackberry Brioche Bread Pudding

Servings: 4-6 Servings
Cooking Time: 30 – 46 Minutes
Ingredients:
- 4 cups brioche bread cubes, loosely packed
- ½ pint blackberries, rinse and pat dry
- 1 cup milk
- 2 eggs
- ½ cup sugar
- 1 teaspoon vanilla
- pinch of salt

Directions:
1. Lightly spray the cooking pot with cooking spray.
2. Place the bread cubes and berries in the pot.
3. In a mixing bowl, whisk remaining ingredients together and pour over the bread and berries.
4. Add the Tender Crisp lid and set to 350 degrees. Bake 45 minutes, or till the pudding puffs up and is starting to brown on top. Serve warm.

229.Chocolate Cheese Cake(1)

Servings: 6 Servings
Cooking Time: 20 Minutes
Ingredients:
- Crust: ¼ cup almond flour
- ¼ cup coconut flour
- 2 Tbsp stevia
- 2 Tbsp melted butter
- Filling: 16 oz cream cheese
- ½ cup baking stevia
- 1/3 cup cocoa powder
- 1 egg and 2 egg yolks
- ¼ cup sour cream
- ¾ cup heavy cream
- 6 oz melted chocolate

- 1 tsp vanilla

Directions:
1. In a small bowl, mix all the ingredients for the crust together. Press the crust into a 7" spring form pan wrapped in foil. Set aside
2. Add the cream cheese, stevia and cocoa powder to a food processor and blend. Add the egg and yolks and blend again. Add remaining ingredients and mix just to combine. Pour cheesecake mix on top of the prepared crust.
3. Place the pan in the Ninja Foodi bowl on top of the metal trivet. Add 2 cups of water to the bowl under the cake. Place the pressure cooker lid on and set it to high pressure for 20 minutes. Allow the pot to naturally release the pressure once he cooking time is done. Chill and then serve.

- **Nutrition Info:** Calories: 474 g, Carbohydrates: 10g , Protein: 8g, Fat: 46 g, Sugar: 4g, Sodium: 338 g

230.Strawberry Chocolate Chip Mug Cake

Servings: 2 Servings
Cooking Time: 10 Minutes
Ingredients:
- 2/3 cup almond flour
- 2 eggs
- 2 Tbsp maple syrup
- 1 tsp vanilla
- 1/8 tsp salt
- ½ cup chopped strawberries
- ¼ cup dark chocolate chips

Directions:
1. Mix all the ingredients together except the strawberries and chocolate chips. Fold well to ensure no lumps.
2. Fold in strawberries and chocolate chips.
3. Pour the batter into two 8 oz mason jars and cover the jars with foil.
4. Place the metal trivet into the Ninja Foodi and add 1 cup of water to the bowl.
5. Place the two mason jars on top of the trivet and close the pressure cooker top. Seal the steamer valve and set the timer to 10 minutes
6. Let the pressure naturally release and then open the lid and enjoy the warm cake.

- **Nutrition Info:** Calories: 326g, Carbohydrates: 35g, Protein: 8g, Fat: 18g, Sugar: 26g, Sodium: 228mg

231. Super Simple Chocolate Brownies

Servings: 6-8 Brownies
Cooking Time: 1-2 Hours
Ingredients:
- 1 ¼ cups semi-sweet chocolate chips
- 1 cup sugar
- 1 cup flour
- ½ cup butter
- 2 eggs + 1 egg yolk, room temperature

Directions:
1. Spray cooker with cooking spray.
2. Melt chocolate chips and butter in a large glass bowl. Add sugar and beat well. Beat in eggs, egg yolk and lastly, flour, just till combined.
3. Pour into cooker. Add lid and select slow cooking on high. Set timer for 1 hour. Brownies are done when batter is set and edges look done. Cool cut into bars.

232. Chocolate Cheese Cake(2)

Servings: 6
Cooking Time: 25 Minutes
Ingredients:
- 2 c. softened cream cheese
- 2 eggs
- 2 tbsps. cocoa powder
- 1 tsp. pure vanilla extract
- ½ c. swerve

Directions:
1. Place eggs, cocoa powder, vanilla extract, swerve and cream cheese in an immersion blender and blend until smooth.
2. Pulse to mix well and transfer the mixture evenly into mason jars.
3. Put the mason jars in the insert of Ninja Foodi and lock the lid.
4. Press "Bake/Roast" and bake for about 15 minutes at 360 degrees F.
5. Place in the refrigerator for 2 hours before serving and serve chilled.
- **Nutrition Info:** 244 calories, 24.8g fat, 2.1g carbs, 4g protein

233. Individual S'mores Pies

Servings: 6 – 12 Pies
Cooking Time: 10 Minutes
Ingredients:
- 2 sheets of puff pastry, thawed
- 2 chocolate bars
- 1 cup mini marshmallows
- ½ cup graham cracker crumbs
- 1 egg, lightly beaten

Directions:
1. Roll out the pastry dough on a lightly floured surface. Cut into 2-3 inch squares, or the size you desire.
2. In the center of half the squares, place a piece of chocolate, some marshmallows and graham crumbs. Moisten the edges of the pastry with water and add the remaining squares on top. Press the edges together. Brush the tops with egg wash.
3. Place 2-3 pies in the air fryer basket at a time, add the Tender Crisp lid and set the temperature to 330 degrees. Bake 5-7 minutes or till the outside is puffed and golden brown. Cool slightly before serving. You can drizzle the tops with melted chocolate or melted marshmallow cream.

234. Coconut Cream Cake

Servings: 8 – 10 Servings
Cooking Time: 35 – 45 Minutes
Ingredients:
- 1 box vanilla cake mix
- 1 box instant coconut pudding
- 1 ½ cups coconut
- 1 cup sour cream
- 1 cup coconut milk, unsweetened
- 4 eggs
- ½ cup coconut oil
- 2 teaspoons coconut extract
- Glaze
- 1 cup powdered sugar
- Enough milk for the desired consistency

Directions:
1. Lightly spray a Bundt cake pan that will fit inside the cooking pot with cooking spray.

2. In a large mixing bowl, beat together all ingredients except the coconut. Stir the coconut in by hand.
3. Pour the batter into the prepared pan and lower into the cooking pot. Add the Tender Crisp lid and set the temperature to 320 degrees. Bake 35 – 40 minutes or till it passes the toothpick test.
4. Carefully remove the cake from the pot and let cool 10 minutes. Transfer to a serving plate.
5. Make the glaze, and toast some additional coconut for garnish. Drizzle the glaze over the cake and top with toasted coconut.

235.Chocolatey 'n Peanut Butter Cakes

Servings: 2
Cooking Time: 15 Minutes
Ingredients:
- 1/2 can black beans, drained and rinsed
- 1/4 cup cocoa powder, unsweetened
- 1/4 cup egg whites
- 2 tbsp canned pumpkin
- 2 tbsp unsweetened applesauce
- 2 tbsp sear button sugar
- 1/2 teaspoon vanilla extract
- ¾ teaspoon baking powder
- ¼ teaspoon salt
- 1 1/2 tablespoon peanut butter baking chips

Directions:
1. Place all the ingredients except the peanut butter chips inside a food processor. Process until smooth.
2. Add the peanut butter chips and fold until evenly distributed within the batter.
3. Place the batter in a ramekin sprayed with cooking oil.
4. Place a steam rack in the Ninja Foodi and add 1 cup water.
5. Place the ramekins with the batter onto the steamer rack.
6. Install pressure lid. Close the lid and press the manual button. Cook on high for 10 minutes.
7. Do natural pressure release.
8. Serve chilled.

- **Nutrition Info:** Calories: 246; carbohydrates: 34.9g; protein: 12.0g; fat: 6.5g

236.Chocolate Pecan Pie

Servings: 8 – 10 Servings
Cooking Time: 35 Minutes
Ingredients:
- 1 pie crust
- 1 cup corn syrup
- 1 cup semisweet chocolate chips
- 1 cup coconut
- 1 cup pecans, chopped
- 3 eggs
- 1/3 cup sugar
- 1/3 cup brown sugar, packed
- 1/3 cup butter, melted
- 1 teaspoon vanilla
- ¼ teaspoon salt

Directions:
1. Unfold the pie crust into a pie plate that fits inside the cooking pot. Place the rack on the bottom of the pot.
2. In a mixing bowl, combine eggs, syrup, sugars, butter, vanilla and salt.
3. Layer the chocolate chips, coconut and pecans on the bottom of the pie crust. Pour the egg mixture evenly on top. Cover the pastry edge with foil and place the pie on the rack in the pot.
4. Add the Tender Crisp lid and set to 350 degrees. Bake 20 minutes then remove the foil and bake another 15 minutes or till set. Carefully remove from the pot and cool completely.

237.Orange-cranberry Pudding

Servings: 2
Cooking Time: 20 Minutes
Ingredients:
- 1/3 cup cranberries
- 1 tablespoon butter, softened
- 1/3 cup sugar
- 1/4 tablespoon vanilla
- 1 orange, juiced and zested
- 1 cup half and half
- 1 1/2 cups brioche, cube
- 2 egg yolks

Directions:

1. In a 6-inch square baking dish, mix well vanilla extract, half & half, orange juice, zest, juice, cranberries, and eggs. Mix thoroughly.
2. Add cubed brioche and toss well to coat in egg mixture. Let it soak for ten minutes. Cover the top with foil.
3. Prepare the Ninja Foodi by placing the inner pot inside.
4. Place wire rack inside and add 2 cups of water.
5. Place baking dish on wire rack.
6. Install pressure lid. Cover and lock lid. Press steam button. Set the timer to 15 minutes.
7. Once done cooking, press stop, and do a quick release.
8. Let it cool completely before serving.
- **Nutrition Info:** Calories: 326; carbohydrates: 48.6g; protein: 5.9g; fat: 12.0g

238.Choco-coffee Cake

Servings: 2
Cooking Time: 25 Minutes
Ingredients:
- 4 tbsp granulated sweetener
- 3 small eggs
- 1/8 teaspoon salt
- 2 tbsp almond flour
- 1 1/4 tablespoons unsweetened cocoa powder
- 1/2 teaspoon vanilla extract
- 1 tablespoon instant coffee crystals
- 2 tbsp heavy cream
- 1-ounce unsweetened chocolate
- 1/4 cup butter
- Coconut oil spray

Directions:

1. Grease sides and bottom of Ninja Foodi with cooking spray.
2. Press sauté button. Add butter and chocolate. Mix well. Make sure to mix constantly so as the bottom doesn't burn. Once fully incorporated, press stop to keep warm.
3. Meanwhile, in a small bowl whisk well vanilla, coffee crystals, and heavy cream.

4. In another bowl, mix well salt, almond flour, and cocoa powder.
5. In a mixing bowl, beat eggs until thick and pale, around 5 minutes while slowly stirring in sweetener.
6. While beating, slowly drizzle and mix in melted butter mixture.
7. Mix in the almond flour mixture and mix well.
8. Add the coffee mixture and beat until fully incorporated.
9. Pour batter into Ninja Foodi.
10. Cover pot, press bake button, and bake for 20 minutes at 350 ºF.
- **Nutrition Info:** Calories: 407; carbohydrates: 27.9g; protein: 3.6g; fat: 31.2g

239.Meyer Lemon Hand Pies

Servings: 6 Servings
Cooking Time: 30 Minutes
Ingredients:
- 1 package refrigerated pie dough
- 1 egg, beaten
- Lemon Curd
- 4 Meyer lemons, juiced
- 8 egg yolks
- 1 ¾ cups sugar
- ½ cup butter, cold and sliced
- 2 tablespoons lemon zest
- Pinch of salt
- Icing
- 1 cup powdered sugar
- ½ lemon

Directions:

1. Place rack in the middle of the cooking pot and add 1-2 inches of water. Set the cooker to sauté on med-high heat and bring to a simmer.
2. Place the yolks and sugar into a bowl that fits inside the pot but is large enough for mixing in, and whisk vigorously till smooth. Add the juice and salt and whisk till smooth again.
3. Once the water reaches a simmer, reduce the heat to med-low and place the bowl on the rack. Cook, whisking constantly, 20-22 minutes, it should be a light yellow color, do

not let it boil. Remove from heat and whisk in the zest.

4. Add butter, one piece at a time, and whisk to combine after each addition. Let cool. Transfer to an airtight container and refrigerate overnight.

5. When ready to make the pies, unfold the pie crust on a lightly floured surface. Roll to a ¼-inch thickness. Use a cookie cutter to cut out 6 circles and place them on a baking sheet. Place 1 tablespoon of the lemon curd in the center of each circle and brush the edges with beaten egg. Fold dough over the filling using a fork to seal the edges. Brush the top of the pies with beaten egg and sprinkle sugar over.

6. Place pies, 2 at a time, in the basket of the air fryer. Add the Tender Crisp lid and set the temperature to 380 degrees. Bake 8-10 minutes, or till golden brown. Let pies cool.

7. Place the powdered sugar in a small bowl and whisk in lemon juice till desired consistency. Drizzle over cooled pies and let sit till the glaze sets. Serve.

240. Scrumptiously Molten Lava Cake

Servings: 3
Cooking Time: 6 Minutes
Ingredients:
- 1 egg
- 4 tablespoon sugar
- 2 tablespoon olive oil
- 4 tablespoon milk
- 4 tablespoon all-purpose flour
- 1 tablespoon cacao powder
- ½ teaspoon baking powder
- Pinch of salt
- Powdered sugar for dusting

Directions:
1. Grease two ramekins with butter or oil. Set aside
2. Pour 1 cup of water in the Ninja Foodi and place the steamer rack.
3. In a medium bowl, mix all the ingredients except the powdered sugar. Blend until well combined.
4. Pour in the ramekins. Place the ramekins in the Ninja Foodi.
5. Install pressure lid and close. Press the pressure button and cook on high for 6 minutes.
6. Once the Ninja Foodi beeps, remove the ramekin.
7. Sprinkle powdered sugar once cooled.
8. Serve and enjoy.
- **Nutrition Info:** Calories: 290; carbohydrates: 30.0g; protein: 5.2g; fat: 16.6g

OTHER FAVORITE RECIPES

241.Baked Beans

Servings: 10 Servings
Cooking Time: 40 Minutes
Ingredients:

- 1 pound dried navy beans, rinsed
- ½ pound bacon, cut into 3-inch pieces
- 2 ½ cups water
- 1 cup onion, chopped
- ½ cup ketchup
- ¼ cup brown sugar
- 2 tablespoons molasses
- 1 teaspoon dry mustard
- ½ teaspoon salt
- ¼ teaspoon pepper

Directions:

1. Add beans to the cooking pot with enough water to cover them completely. Secure the lid and select pressure cooking on high. Cook for 1 minute, then let rest for one hour. Drain and rinse the beans and discard any that are floating.
2. Set the cooker to sauté on med-high heat. Add the bacon and cook till crisp. Transfer the bacon to a paper towel lined plate and set aside.
3. Add the onion and cook till tender, scraping up the brown bits on the bottom of the pot.
4. Add all of the ingredients, except the bacon to the onions and stir to combine. Set the cooker back to pressure cooking on high and cook 35 minutes.
5. When the timer goes off wait 10 minutes, then use quick release to remove the lid. Check to see if the beans are tender, if not cook a few minutes longer.
6. Set the cooker back to sauté on medium heat and stir in the bacon. Cook, stirring often, till sauce thickens to desired consistency. Serve or store in the refrigerator.

242.Southwest Chicken Egg Rolls

Servings: 6 Pieces
Cooking Time: 20 Minutes
Ingredients:

- 6 egg roll wrappers
- 1 cup Mexican blend cheese, grated
- ½ cup chicken, cooked and shredded
- ½ cup red onion, chopped fine
- ½ cup bell pepper, chopped fine
- ½ cup fire roasted tomatoes, drained
- ½ avocado, chopped fine
- 1 teaspoon chili powder
- 1 teaspoon olive oil
- Water

Directions:

1. Set cooker to saute setting on med-high heat. Add olive oil and red onion. Cook, stirring frequently till onion becomes translucent.
2. Add bell peppers and cook 2-3 minutes. Add tomatoes and cook an additional 2-3 minutes, stirring frequently.
3. Transfer vegetables to a bowl and mix in the remaining ingredients till blended.
4. Place wrappers on a work surface. Place about 2 tablespoons of filling near one corner. Fold the corner closest to the filling over it. Fold both side corners toward the center and roll it up. Seal with water. Lightly spray the rolls with cooking spray on both sides.
5. Wipe out the cooker. Lightly spray the rack with cooking spray and place it into the pot. Place egg rolls on the rack and lock the Tender Crisp lid in place.
6. Set the temperature for 375 degrees and cook egg rolls for 8 minutes. Flip them over and cook another 8 minutes or till golden brown.

243.Zucchini Pasta With Walnuts & Basil

Servings: 3 – 4 Servings
Cooking Time: 10 Minutes
Ingredients:

- 4 large zucchini, peeled
- ½ cup walnuts, chopped
- 1/3 cup bacon grease
- ¼ cup fresh basil, chopped
- 2 cloves garlic, chopped fine
- 2 teaspoons salt

Directions:

1. If you have a vegetable spiralizer, use it to create zucchini noodles. If you don't, cut the zucchini, lengthwise into long, thin strips that resemble spaghetti noodles. Place in a colander and sprinkle with salt, toss to coat. Place over the kitchen sink for 1 hour to extract the water.
2. Rinse the zucchini thoroughly till no salt remains. Drain on paper towels.
3. Set the cooker to saute on med-high heat and add the bacon grease. Once it is hot, add garlic and zucchini and cook, stirring often, about 4-5 minutes or it is al dente.
4. Stir in basil and walnuts and cook another 2 minutes. Serve.

244.Easy Chow Mein Topped With Green Onions

Servings: 2
Cooking Time: 15 Minutes
Ingredients:
- 4 oz chow mein noodles
- 2 tablespoons peanut oil
- 4 green onions, chopped, white and green parts separated
- 3 cloves garlic, minced
- 1 teaspoon ginger , minced
- 1 small bell pepper, thinly sliced
- Sauce ingredients:
- 1/4 cup chicken broth
- 2 tablespoons shaoxing wine , or dry sherry
- 2 tablespoons oyster sauce
- 1 tablespoon soy sauce
- 1/2 teaspoon sesame oil

Directions:
1. In a small bowl, whisk well all sauce ingredients.
2. Boil noodles according to package instructions. Pour into colander and run under tap water to stop the cooking process. Drain well.
3. In Ninja Foodi, press sauté button and heat 3 tbsps oil. Heat for 4 minutes. Once hot add noodles and cook for a minute.
4. Stir in ginger and garlic. Cook for a minute until fragrant.
5. Stir in bell pepper and cook for 2 minutes.
6. Add sauce and toss noodles to coat well.

7. Serve and enjoy.
- **Nutrition Info:** Calories: 441; carbohydrates: 49.9g; protein: 6.6g; fat: 23.8g

245.Olive-brined Air Fryer Turkey Breasts

Servings: 7
Cooking Time: 45 Minutes
Ingredients:
- ½ cup salt
- 6 cups water
- ½ cup butter milk
- 3 ½ pounds boneless turkey breasts
- 1 sprig rosemary
- 2 sprigs thyme

Directions:
1. Place all ingredients in a large bowl or stock pot and allow the turkey to soak in the brine for at least 24 hours.
2. Rinse the turkey and pat dry.
3. Place in the ceramic pot the FoodiTM Cook & CrispTM basket
4. Place the turkey breasts in the basket.
5. Close the crisping lid and press the Air Crisp button before pressing the START button.
6. Adjust the cooking time to 45 minutes.
- **Nutrition Info:** Calories: 135; Carbohydrates: 1.4g; Protein: 30.2g; Fat: 0.9g; Sugar:0 g; Sodium: 62mg

246.Easy Crab Wontons

Servings: 16 Pieces
Cooking Time: 10 Minutes
Ingredients:
- 16 wonton wrappers
- ¾ cup lump crab meat
- 2 green onions, chopped
- 3 tablespoons cream cheese, soft
- Black pepper
- Old Bay seasoning

Directions:
1. Combine all ingredients in a mixing bowl and mix well
2. Lay out wrappers on a work surface. Moisten with a dab of water and spoon about 1 ½ teaspoons filling on each.
3. Pull two opposite corners up over filling and pinch together. Repeat with other

corners. Spray the wontons lightly with cooking spray.

4. Spray the cooking pot with and add the wontons, you will have to cook them in batches.
5. Lock the Tender Crisp lid in place and set temperature to 350 degrees. Cook 8 minutes or till they are golden brown and crisp.
6. Serve with your favorite dipping sauce or enjoy them on their own.

247.Rum Spiced Nuts

Servings: 3 Cups
Cooking Time: 10 Minutes
Ingredients:
- 3 cups mixed nuts
- 2 tablespoons butter
- 2 tablespoons dark rum
- 2 tablespoons sugar
- 1 tablespoon salt
- 2 teaspoons curry powder
- 1 teaspoon ancho chile powder
- 1 teaspoon cinnamon
- 1 teaspoon cumin

Directions:
1. Set the cooker to sauté on medium heat. Add nuts and cook to lightly toast them, about 3-5 minutes, stirring frequently.
2. Add the butter and rum to the nuts and cook, stirring frequently, till most of the liquid evaporates and the nuts are glassy.
3. In a large bowl, add remaining ingredients and stir to combine. Add the glazed nuts and toss well to coat.
4. Dump the nuts onto a large baking sheet to cool. Serve immediately or store in an airtight container.

248.Spicy Pressure Cooker Short Ribs

Servings: 4
Cooking Time: 45 Minutes
Ingredients:
- 1 habanero pepper, minced
- 1 ½ teaspoons black pepper
- 1 teaspoon paprika
- ½ teaspoon ground cumin
- 2 pounds beef short ribs

- 1 can cola
- 2 tablespoons apple cider vinegar
- 1 tablespoon raspberry jam
- 1 tablespoon Worcestershire sauce
- 1 tablespoon brown sugar
- 2 teaspoons canola oil
- ½ onion, diced
- 4 cloves of garlic, minced
- 2 tablespoons water
- 2 tablespoons cornstarch

Directions:
1. In a Ziploc bag, place the habanero, black pepper, paprika, cumin, beef short ribs, cola, apple cider vinegar, raspberry jam, Worcestershire sauce, and sugar. Marinate for at least 2 hours in the fridge.
2. Press the Sear/Sauté button and press the START button.
3. Heat the olive oil and sauté the onion and garlic until fragrant. Stir in the marinated beef (liquid included) and adjust the moisture.
4. Place the pressure lid and set the vent to the SEAL position. Press the Pressure button.
5. Adjust the cooking time to 45 minutes.
6. Once cooking is done, do natural pressure release to open the lid.
7. Open the lid and press the Sear/Sauté button and stir in the cornstarch slurry.
8. Allow to simmer until the sauce thickens.
- **Nutrition Info:** Calories: 582; Carbohydrates: 24.1g; Protein: 22g; Fat: 44.1g; Sugar: 10.4g; Sodium: 224mg

249.Pressure Cooker Bone-in Pork Chops With Vegetables

Servings:4
Cooking Time: 30 Minutes
Ingredients:
- 4 ¾ -inch bone-in pork chops
- Salt and pepper to taste
- ¼ cup butter, divided
- 1 cup baby carrots
- 4 whole potatoes, peeled and halved
- 1 onion, chopped
- 1 cup vegetable broth
- 3 tablespoons Worcestershire sauce

Directions:

1. Season the beef with salt and pepper. Dredge in flour.
2. Press the Sear/Sauté button and then the START button.
3. Season the pork with salt and pepper to taste.
4. Put half of the butter in the pot and sear the pork for at least 2 minutes on both sides.
5. Stir in the carrots, potatoes, onions, vegetable broth, and Worcestershire sauce.
6. Close the pressure lid and set the vent to SEAL.
7. Press the Pressure button and adjust the cooking time to 30 minutes.
8. Do natural pressure release.
9. Once the lid is open, stir in the remaining butter.
- **Nutrition Info:** Calories: 577; Carbohydrates: 60.3g; Protein: 34.6g; Fat: 21.9g; Sugar: 20.6g; Sodium: 404mg

250.Ninja Foodie Short Ribs

Servings: 8
Cooking Time: 60 Minutes
Ingredients:

- 1 bottle (750mL) red wine
- 4 pounds beef short ribs
- 3 tablespoons unsalted butter
- 1 ½ cups onion, chopped
- 3 cloves of garlic, minced
- 1 cup minced carrots
- 2 sprigs fresh rosemary
- 2 cups chicken stock
- Salt and pepper to taste

Directions:

1. Place all ingredients in the pot except for the hard-boiled eggs.
2. Close the pressure lid and set the vent to SEAL.
3. Press the Pressure button and adjust the cooking time to 60 minutes.
4. Do natural pressure release.
- **Nutrition Info:** Calories: 436; Carbohydrates: 13.2g; Protein: 15.9g; Fat: 35.5g; Sugar: 5.8g; Sodium: 277mg On

251.Chinese Style Steamed Fish

Servings: 3
Cooking Time: 25 Minutes
Ingredients:

- 1 ½ pounds halibut, cut into 4 pieces
- 3 green onions, chopped
- 2 fresh mushrooms, sliced
- 6 leaves napa cabbage, slice
- 2 slices fresh ginger root, chopped
- 2 clove of garlic, chopped
- ¼ cup soy sauce
- 1/8 cup water
- ¼ cup crushed red pepper flakes
- ½ cup fresh cilantro sprigs for garnish

Directions:

1. Place the FoodiTM Cook &CrispTM reversible rack inside the ceramic pot.
2. Pour water into the pot.
3. In a big aluminum foil, place the halibut and arrange the rest of the ingredients on top of the halibuts.
4. Fold the aluminum foil and crimp the edges.
5. Place on the reversible rack.
6. Close the pressure lid and set the vent to SEAL.
7. Press the Steam button and adjust the cooking time to 25 minutes.
- **Nutrition Info:** Calories: 210; Carbohydrates: 5.2g; Protein: 37.7g; Fat: 4.2g; Sugar: 2.1g; Sodium: 636mg

252.Zucchini Cream Cheese Fries

Servings: 4
Cooking Time: 20 Minutes
Ingredients:

- 1 lb. zucchini, sliced
- Salt
- 1 c. cream cheese
- 2 tbsps. olive oil

Directions:

1. Put zucchini in a colander and add salt and cream cheese.
2. Put oil and zucchini in the pot of Ninja Foodi and lock the lid.
3. Press "Air Crisp" and set the timer to 10 minutes at 365 degrees F.
4. Dish out from the Ninja Foodi and serve.

- **Nutrition Info:** 374 calories, 36.6g fat, 7.1g carbs, 7.7g protein

253.Crunchy Tortilla Chips

Servings: 6
Cooking Time: 3 Minutes
Ingredients:
- 8 corn tortillas, cut into triangle
- 1 tbsp. olive oil
- Salt, to taste

Directions:
1. Coat the tortilla chips pieces with oil evenly.
2. Arrange the "Cook & Crisp Basket" in the pot of Ninja Foodi.
3. Close the Ninja Foodi with crisping lid and select "Air Crisp".
4. Press "Start/Stop" to begin and set the temperature to 390 degrees F.
5. Set the time for 5 minutes to preheat.
6. Now, place the tortilla chips pieces into "Cook & Crisp Basket".
7. Close the Ninja Foodi with crisping lid and select "Air Crisp".
8. Set the temperature to 390 degrees F for 3 minutes.
9. Press "Start/Stop" to begin.
10. Open the lid and serve warm.
- **Nutrition Info:** Calories per serving: 90; Carbohydrates: 14.3g; Protein: 1.8g; Fat: 3.2g; Sugar: 0.3g; Sodium: 42mg; Fiber: 2g

254.Spicy Honey Mustard Pork Roast

Servings: 6
Cooking Time: 1 Hour And 30 Minutes
Ingredients:
- 3 pounds pork roast
- ¼ cup honey
- 2 tablespoons Dijon mustard
- 2 tablespoons black pepper
- ½ teaspoon salt
- ½ teaspoon dried thyme

Directions:
1. Place in the ceramic pot the FoodiTM Cook & CrispTM reversible rack.
2. Score the pork roast with a knife and place on a circular baking dish that will fit in the Ninja Foodi.
3. In a mixing bowl, mix together the rest of the ingredients until well-blended.
4. Brush the pork with the spice rub.
5. Place the pork in a baking dish on the rack.
6. Close the crisping lid and press the Bake/Roast button before pressing the START button.
7. Adjust the cooking time to 1hour and 30 minutes.
- **Nutrition Info:** Calories: 242; Carbohydrates: 14.1g; Protein: 26.5g; Fat: 8.8g; Sugar: 7.9g; Sodium: 366mg

255.Buttery Corn

Servings: 2
Cooking Time: 20 Minutes
Ingredients:
- 2 ears corn on the cob
- Salt and freshly ground pepper, to taste
- 2 tbsp. butter, softened and divided

Directions:
1. Season the corn with salt and black pepper and then, rub with half of butter.
2. Arrange the "Cook & Crisp Basket" in the pot of Ninja Foodi.
3. Close the Ninja Foodi with crisping lid and select "Air Crisp".
4. Press "Start/Stop" to begin and set the temperature to 320 degrees F.
5. Set the time for 5 minutes to preheat.
6. With a piece of foil, wrap each cob and place into "Cook & Crisp Basket".
7. Close the Ninja Foodi with crisping lid and select "Air Crisp".
8. Set the temperature to 320 degrees F for 20 minutes.
9. Press "Start/Stop" to begin.
10. Open the lid and transfer the cobs into a bowl.
11. Coat with the remaining butter and serve.
- **Nutrition Info:** Calories per serving: 234; Carbohydrates: 29g; Protein: 5.1g; Fat: 13.3g; Sugar: 5g; Sodium: 182mg; Fiber: 4.2g

256.Cheesy Shepherd's Pie

Servings: 6 Servings
Cooking Time: 30 Minutes

Ingredients:

- 1 pound ground beef
- 3 medium russet potatoes, peeled and cut into 1-inch cubes
- 3 carrot, chopped
- 1 cup onion, chopped fine
- 1 cup mushrooms, chopped
- 1 cup peas, frozen
- 1 cup water
- 1 cup beef broth
- 1 cup cheddar cheese, grated
- 1 egg
- 2 tablespoons butter
- 2 tablespoons Worcestershire
- 2 tablespoons flour
- 1 ½ teaspoons salt
- 1 teaspoon garlic powder
- 1 teaspoon pepper

Directions:

1. Add potatoes and water to cooking pot. Secure lid and select pressure cooking on high. Set timer for 8 minutes. When the timer goes off, drain the potatoes and place them in a large mixing bowl.
2. Add the egg, garlic powder, ½ teaspoon salt and butter and blend together with a hand mixer. Set aside.
3. Set the cooker to sauté on med-high heat and add the ground beef. Cook, stirring often, till no longer pink. Drain the grease. Add Worcestershire, vegetables, salt and pepper and stir to combine.
4. In a small measuring cup, stir the flour and broth together then add to beef mixture. Cook, stirring often, about 3 minutes or till sauce begins to thicken. Transfer to a baking dish that will fit inside the cooking pot.
5. Top the beef mixture with the mashed potatoes in an even layer. Cover the dish with foil.
6. Rinse out the cooking pot and add the rack to it. Add ½ cups water then place the baking dish on the rack. Secure the lid and select pressure cooking on high. Set the timer for 10 minutes.
7. Use quick release to remove the lid. Carefully remove the dish from the pot,

unless you are going to broil the top. Remove the foil and sprinkle the cheese on top. Let rest for 10 minutes before serving.

257.Flaky Fish With Ginger

Servings: 2
Cooking Time: 15minutes
Ingredients:

- 1 pound halibut fillet, skin removed
- 1 teaspoon salt to taste
- 1 tablespoon fresh ginger, sliced thinly
- 3 tablespoons green onion
- 1 tablespoon dark soy sauce
- 1 tablespoon peanut oil
- 2 teaspoons sesame oil

Directions:

1. Place the FoodiTM Cook &CrispTM reversible rack inside the ceramic pot.
2. Pour a cup of water in the pot.
3. Season the halibut fillets with salt to taste.
4. Place in a heat-proof ceramic dish. Drizzle with the rest of the ingredients.
5. Place the ceramic dish with the fish inside on the reversible rack.
6. Close the pressure lid and set the vent to SEAL.
7. Press the Steam button and adjust the cooking time to 15 minutes.
8. Do quick pressure release.
- **Nutrition Info:** Calories: 352; Carbohydrates: 2g; Protein: 48.1g; Fat: 16.8g; Sugar: 0.2g; Sodium: 1908mg

258.Juicy Asian Steamed Chicken

Servings: 4
Cooking Time: 45 Minutes
Ingredients:

- 4 bone-in chicken thighs
- 1 teaspoon salt
- 1 piece fresh ginger, sliced
- 3 green onions, sliced
- 2 cloves of garlic, minced
- 1 ½ tablespoons fish sauce
- 1 tablespoon vinegar
- 1 tablespoon lime juice
- 4 Thai green chilies, chopped
- 5 sprigs, cilantro, chopped
- 1 teaspoon sugar

Directions:
1. Place all ingredients in a Ziploc bag and allow to marinate in the fridge for at least 2 hours.
2. Place the FoodiTM Cook &CrispTM reversible rack inside the ceramic pot.
3. Pour water into the pot.
4. Place the marinated chicken on the reversible rack.
5. Close the pressure lid and set the vent to SEAL.
6. Press the Steam button and adjust the cooking time to 45 minutes.
- **Nutrition Info:** Calories: 314; Carbohydrates: 19.2g; Protein: 19.9g; Fat:17.3 g; Sugar: 10.5g; Sodium: 935mg

259.Balsamic Roasted Pork Loin

Servings: 4
Cooking Time: 1 Hour And 30 Minutes
Ingredients:
- 2 tablespoons steak seasoning rub
- ½ cup balsamic vinegar
- ½ cup olive oil
- 2 pounds boneless pork loin roast

Directions:
1. Place in the ceramic pot the FoodiTM Cook &CrispTM reversible rack.
2. Mix the steak seasoning rub, balsamic vinegar, and olive oil.
3. Rub the pork loin roast with the seasoning.
4. Close the crisping lid and press the Bake/Roast button before pressing the START button.
5. Adjust the cooking time to 1 hour and 30 minutes.
- **Nutrition Info:** Calories: 297; Carbohydrates: 3.1g; Protein: 18.3g; Fat: 23.4g; Sugar: 0.8g; Sodium:732 mg

260.Steamed Brisket In Guinness

Servings: 8
Cooking Time: 50 Minutes
Ingredients:
- 3 ½ cups Irish stout beer (Guinness)
- 2 bay leaves
- 1 tablespoon salt
- 1 tablespoon ground black pepper
- 2 teaspoons paprika
- 1 teaspoon dried basil
- 1 teaspoon dried oregano
- 1 teaspoon garlic powder
- 1 teaspoon onion powder
- 4 pounds beef brisket
- 2 large onions, sliced
- 2 tablespoons cornstarch
- 3 tablespoons water

Directions:
1. Place the FoodiTM Cook &CrispTM reversible rack inside the ceramic pot.
2. Pour the Guinness in the pot. Stir in the bay leaves.
3. In a small bowl, combine the salt, black pepper, paprika, dried basil, oregano, garlic powder, and onion powder. This will be the dry rub.
4. Season the beef brisket with the dry rub. Place the beef brisket on the reversible rack.
5. Close the pressure lid and set the vent to SEAL.
6. Press the Steam button and adjust the cooking time to 50 minutes.
7. Do quick pressure release. Once the lid is open, remove the beef. Take out the basket as well. Press the Sear/Sauté button and allow the sauce to simmer.
8. Stir in the onions and cornstarch until the sauce thickens.
9. Pour the sauce over the steamed beef.
- **Nutrition Info:** Calories: 714; Carbohydrates: 83.4g; Protein: 46.2g; Fat: 21.7g; Sugar: 0.9g; Sodium: 693mg

261.Tasty 'n Easy To Make Baked Potatoes

Servings: 2
Cooking Time: 35 Minutes
Ingredients:
- 2 medium russet potato
- 2 teaspoon canola oil
- 1/2 teaspoon onion powder
- Salt and pepper to taste
- 2 tablespoons cream cheese
- 2 tablespoons chopped chives

Directions:
1. Brush the potatoes until clean.

2. Place the Cook & Crisp basket in the Ninja Foodi and add potatoes.
3. Brush with oil on all surface and season with onion powder, salt, and pepper.
4. Close the Ninja Foodi and cook for 35 minutes at 350 ºF.
5. Once cooked, slice through the potato and serve with cream cheese and chives.
- **Nutrition Info:** Calories: 413; carbs: 72.3g; protein:10.2 g; fat: 9.2g

262.Lemon Pepper Wings

Servings: 4 Servings
Cooking Time: 20 Minutes
Ingredients:
- 2 ½ pounds chicken wing pieces
- 1 cup flour
- 1/3 cup butter
- 1 teaspoon lemon pepper
- ½ teaspoon salt
- ½ teaspoon black pepper

Directions:
1. Mix flour with salt in pepper in a large bowl. Add wing pieces, in small batches to flour and toss to coat each piece well.
2. Spray the fryer basket lightly with cooking spray. Add wings, in batches, to basket and place in the cooker. Lock the Tender Crisp lid in place and set temperature to 360 degrees.
3. Cook for 10 minutes, then turn the wings over and cook an additional 10 minutes or till they are golden brown.
4. Place the butter in a medium mixing bowl and melt in the microwave. Stir in the lemon pepper seasoning and then add cooked wings and toss to coat.
5. Serve with your favorite dipping sauce.

263.Chinese Pork Roast

Servings: 8
Cooking Time: 1 Hour And 30 Minutes
Ingredients:
- 4 pounds pork roast, trimmed
- ¾ cup soy sauce
- ½ cup dry sherry
- 1/3 cup honey
- 2 cloves of garlic, minced

- ½ teaspoon ground ginger

Directions:
1. Place in the ceramic pot the FoodiTM Cook &CrispTM reversible rack.
2. Place all ingredients in a bowl and allow the meat to marinate in the fridge for at least 12 hours.
3. Place the marinated meat on the rack.
4. Close the crisping lid and press the Bake/Roast button before pressing the START button.
5. Adjust the cooking time to 1 hour and 30 minutes.
6. Meanwhile, put the marinade in a saucepan and bring to a simmer until the sauce has reduced.
7. Halfway through the cooking time, baste the pork with sauce.
- **Nutrition Info:** Calories: 345; Carbohydrates: 15.1g; Protein: 22.3g; Fat: 21.5g; Sugar: 8.6g; Sodium: 1310mg

264.Coconut Carrots

Servings: 4 Servings
Cooking Time: 16 Minutes
Ingredients:
- 4 cups sliced carrots
- 2 Tablespoons coconut oil
- 1 tsp salt
- ½ tsp pepper

Directions:
1. Cut the carrots in half and toss together with the coconut oil, salt and pepper.
2. Place the cook and crisp pot inside the Ninja Foodi. Close the crisper lid and set the pot to 400 degrees F using the air crisp function.
3. Add the carrots to the basket and set the timer for 8 minutes.
4. Open the lid, mix the carrots inside the pot and then cook for another 8 minutes to get nice and crispy.
- **Nutrition Info:** Calories: 113g, Carbohydrates: 12g, Protein: 1g, Fat: 7g, Sugar: 6g, Sodium: 122mg

265.Ninja Foodi Baked Fudge

Servings:6
Cooking Time: 50 Minutes

Ingredients:

- 2 cups white sugar
- ½ cup all-purpose flour
- ½ cup cocoa powder
- 4 eggs, beaten
- 1 cup butter, melted
- 2 teaspoons vanilla extract
- 1 cup chopped pecans

Directions:

1. Place in the ceramic pot the FoodiTM Cook &CrispTM reversible rack.
2. Close the crisping lid and press the Broil button before pressing the START button to preheat the Ninja Foodi.
3. In a bowl, sift together the sugar, flour, and cocoa. Add in eggs, melted butter, vanilla, and pecans. Mix to combine everything.
4. Pour the batter into a baking pan that will fit inside the Ninja Foodi.
5. Place in the preheated Ninja Foodi and close the crisping lid.
6. Press the Bake/Roast button before pressing the START button.
7. Adjust the cooking time to 50 minutes.
- **Nutrition Info:** Calories: 397; Carbohydrates: 40.7g; Protein: 4.3g; Fat: 24.1g; Sugar: 25.3g; Sodium: 159mg

266.Chinese Steamed Fish

Servings: 2
Cooking Time: 10 Minutes
Ingredients:

- 1 pound red snapper fillets
- 1 tablespoon grated ginger
- 1 tablespoon soy sauce
- 2 tablespoons sesame oil
- 2 shiitake mushrooms, sliced thinly
- 1 tomato, quartered
- ½ fresh red chili pepper, chopped
- 2 sprigs of cilantro, chopped
- Salt and pepper to taste

Directions:

1. Place the FoodiTM Cook &CrispTM reversible rack inside the ceramic pot.
2. Pour a cup of water in the pot.
3. One a heat-proof ceramic bowl, place the fish and season with salt, pepper, ginger, and soy sauce.

4. Pour over sesame oil and add mushrooms, tomatoes, and red chili on top.
5. Place the ceramic dish with the fish on the reversible rack.
6. Close the pressure lid and set the vent to SEAL.
7. Press the Steam button and adjust the cooking time to 10 minutes.
8. Do quick pressure release.
9. Serve with chopped cilantro
- **Nutrition Info:** Calories: 290; Carbohydrates: 5.9g; Protein: 48.3g; Fat: 8.1g; Sugar: 0.8g; Sodium: 1187mg

267.Chinese Steamed Buns

Servings: 8
Cooking Time: 30 Minutes
Ingredients:

- 1 tablespoon active dry yeast
- 1 teaspoon white sugar
- ¼ cup all-purpose flour
- ¼ cup warm water
- ½ cup water
- 1 ½ cups all-purpose flour
- ¼ teaspoon salt
- 2 tablespoons white sugar
- 1 tablespoon vegetable oil
- ½ teaspoon baking powder

Directions:

1. Place the FoodiTM Cook &CrispTM reversible rack inside the ceramic pot. Pour water into the pot.
2. In a mixing bowl, mix together the dry yeast, white sugar, ¼ cup all-purpose flour, and ¼ cup water. Allow the yeast to activate for 10 minutes. This is evident with bubbles forming on top.
3. In another bowl, combine ½ cup water, 1 ½ cups all-purpose flour, salt, white sugar, vegetable oil, and baking powder. Add in the activated yeast mixture.
4. Fold the mixture until you form a dough.
5. On a floured surface, pour the dough and knead for at least 10 minutes using your hands until it becomes springy. Cover the bowl with warm towel and allow to rest for 2 hours.

6. Once risen, knead the dough and cut into 8 equal parts. Cover with warm towel and allow to rest for another 2 hours.
7. Place on the reversible rack. Close the pressure lid and set the vent to SEAL.
8. Press the Steam button and adjust the cooking time to 30 minutes.
- **Nutrition Info:** Calories: 44; Carbohydrates: 8.4g; Protein: 1.1g; Fat:0.6 g; Sugar:1.4 g; Sodium: 35mg

268.Unique Apple Pastries

Servings: 8
Cooking Time: 10 Minutes
Ingredients:
- ½ large apple, peeled, cored and chopped
- 1 tsp. fresh orange zest, grated finely
- ½ tbsp. white sugar
- ½ tsp. ground cinnamon
- 7.05-oz. prepared frozen puff pastry

Directions:
1. In a bowl, mix together all ingredients except puff pastry.
2. Cut the pastry in 16 squares.
3. Place about a tsp. of the apple mixture in the center of each square.
4. Fold each square into a triangle and press the edges slightly with wet fingers.
5. Then with a fork, press the edges firmly.
6. Arrange the "Cook & Crisp Basket" in the pot of Ninja Foodi.
7. Close the Ninja Foodi with crisping lid and select "Air Crisp".
8. Press "Start/Stop" to begin and set the temperature to 390 degrees F.
9. Set the time for 5 minutes to preheat.
10. Now, place the pastries into "Cook & Crisp Basket".
11. Close the Ninja Foodi with crisping lid and select "Air Crisp".
12. Set the temperature to 390 degrees F for 10 minutes.
13. Press "Start/Stop" to begin.
14. Open the lid and serve warm.
- **Nutrition Info:** Calories per serving: 119; Carbohydrates: 11.3g; Protein: 1.5g; Fat: 7.6g; Sugar: 1.9g; Sodium: 50mg; Fiber: 0.7g

269.Pumpkin & Bacon Risotto

Servings: 6 Servings
Cooking Time: 1 Hour
Ingredients:
- 4 ½ cups chicken broth
- 6 strips bacon, chopped
- 1 ½ cups onion, chopped
- 1 cup Arborio rice, uncooked
- ½ cup Parmesan cheese
- ¼ cup pumpkin puree
- 2 tablespoons parsley, chopped
- 1 tablespoon olive oil
- salt and black pepper

Directions:
1. Set cooker to sauté on med-high heat and add oil. When the oil is hot, add bacon and onions and cook till onions are tender and bacon starts to crisp, about 15 minutes.
2. Add the rice, salt and pepper. Cook, stirring often, 5 minutes. Stir in broth and cook another 10 minutes.
3. Reduce the heat to low and cover. Cook 25 minutes, or till rice is done. Stir the pumpkin in during the last 5 minutes of cooking.
4. Turn the heat up to med-high and stir in the cheese. Cook, uncovered, till most of the liquid is gone. Serve immediately garnished with the chopped parsley and additional Parmesan cheese.

270.Heart-felt Caramelized Onions

Servings: 4
Cooking Time: 65 Minutes
Ingredients:
- 2 tbsps. butter, unsalted
- 3 sliced onions
- 2 tbsps. water
- 1 tsp. salt

Directions:
1. Set your pot to Sauté mode and adjust the heat to Medium, pre-heat the inner pot for 5 minutes
2. Add butter and melt, add water, salt, onions, and stir well
3. Lock pressure lid into place, making sure that the pressure valve is locked
4. Cook on HIGH pressure for 30 minutes

5. Quick release the pressure once done
6. Remove the lid and set the pot to Sauté mode, let it sear in the Medium-HIGH mode for about 15 minutes until the liquid is almost gone
7. Enjoy!
- **Nutrition Info:** 110 calories, 6g fat, 14g carbs, 2g protein

271.Pressure Cooker Pasta Stew

Servings:6
Cooking Time: 20 Minutes
Ingredients:
- 1 pound lean ground beef
- 1 cloves of garlic, minced
- 1 onion, chopped
- 1 package bow tie pasta
- 1 can tomato sauce
- 1 can stewed tomatoes
- 1 teaspoon oregano
- 1 teaspoon Italian seasoning
- 1 cup mozzarella cheese
- 1 cup ricotta cheese
- Salt and pepper to taste

Directions:
1. Season the beef with salt and pepper. Dredge in flour.
2. Press the Sear/Sauté button and then the START button.
3. Sauté the beef until some of the fat has rendered. Stir in the garlic and onions until fragrant.
4. Add in the pasta, tomatoes, oregano, and Italian seasoning. Season with salt and pepper to taste. Stir in the rest of the ingredients.
5. Close the pressure lid and set the vent to SEAL.
6. Press the Pressure button and adjust the cooking time to 10 minutes.
7. Do quick pressure release.
8. Once the lid is open, press the Sear/Sauté button then the START button.
9. Stir in the cheese and allow to simmer for another 5 minutes.
- **Nutrition Info:** Calories: 469; Carbohydrates: 53g; Protein: 29.3g; Fat: 15.5g; Sugar: 24.3g; Sodium: 567mg

272.Ninja Foodi Chili

Servings:4
Cooking Time: 30 Minutes
Ingredients:
- 2 tablespoons olive oil
- 1 onion, chopped
- 2 cloves of garlic, minced
- 2 pound ground beef
- 1 green bell pepper, chopped
- 1 jalapeno pepper, chopped
- 2 cans red kidney beans, rinsed and drained
- 2 cans diced tomatoes, undrained
- 3 tablespoons tomato paste
- 1 tablespoon sugar
- 2 teaspoons unsweetened cocoa powder
- ¼ teaspoon crushed red pepper flakes
- 2 tablespoons chili powder
- 2 teaspoons ground cumin
- ½ teaspoon salt
- 2 cups water

Directions:
1. Press the Sear/Sauté button and then the START button.
2. Heat the oil and sauté the garlic and onion until fragrant.
3. Stir in the ground beef and cook for another 2 minutes.
4. Add in the rest of the ingredients.
5. Close the pressure lid and set the vent to SEAL.
6. Press the Pressure button and adjust the cooking time to 30 minutes.
- **Nutrition Info:** Calories: 285; Carbohydrates: 35.3g; Protein: 22.3g; Fat: 14.9g; Sugar: 13.8g; Sodium: 790mg

273.Spiced Roasted Broccoli

Servings:2
Cooking Time: 20 Minutes
Ingredients:
- 2 cups broccoli florets
- 1 yellow bell pepper, sliced
- 1 teaspoon garlic powder
- 1 tablespoon steak seasoning
- 2 teaspoons chili powder
- 1 tablespoon extra-virgin olive oil
- Salt and pepper to taste

Directions:

1. Place in the ceramic pot the FoodiTM Cook &CrispTM basket insert.
2. Toss all ingredients in a mixing bowl.
3. Place the vegetables in the basket.
4. Close the crisping lid and press the Bake/Roast button before pressing the START button.
5. Adjust the cooking time to 20 minutes.
6. Give the basket a shake to roast the vegetables evenly
- **Nutrition Info:** Calories: 76; Carbohydrates: 8g; Protein: 2.1g; Fat: 3.9g; Sugar: 0.6g; Sodium: 718mg

274.Great Snacking Nuts

Servings: 20
Cooking Time: 14 Minutes
Ingredients:
- ½ C. unsalted butter
- 1½ C. walnuts
- 1½ C. cashews
- 3 tsp. ground cinnamon
- ½ C. powdered sugar

Directions:

1. Select "Sauté/Sear" setting of Ninja Foodi and place the butter into the pot.
2. Press "Start/Stop" to begin and heat for about 2-3 minutes.
3. Add the nuts and cook, uncovered for about 15 minutes.
4. Press "Start/Stop" to stop the cooking and stir in the cinnamon and sugar.
5. Close the crisping lid and select "Slow Cooker".
6. Set on "High" for about 2-2½ hours.
7. Press "Start/Stop" to begin.
8. Open the lid and transfer the nuts into a bowl to cool before serving.
- **Nutrition Info:** Calories per serving: 170; Carbohydrates: 7.6g; Protein: 3.9g; Fat: 14.9g; Sugar: 3.6g; Sodium: 35mg; Fiber: 1.1g

275.Brekky Bacon 'n Egg Risotto

Servings: 2
Cooking Time: 10 Minutes
Ingredients:
- 1 1/2 cups chicken broth
- 1/3 cup chopped onion
- 2 eggs
- 2 tablespoons grated parmesan cheese
- 3 slices center cut bacon, chopped
- 3 tablespoons dry white wine
- 3/4 cup arborio rice
- Chives, for garnish
- Salt and pepper, to taste

Directions:

1. Press sauté button and cook bacon to a crisp, around 6 minutes.
2. Stir in onion and sauté for 3 minutes. Add rice and sauté for a minute.
3. Pour in wine and deglaze pot. Continue sautéing until wine is completely absorbed by rice, around 5 minutes.
4. Stir in chicken broth.
5. Install pressure lid. Close Ninja Foodi, press pressure button, choose high settings, and set time to 5 minutes.
6. Meanwhile, cook eggs sunny side up to desired doneness.
7. Once done cooking, do a quick release. Stir in pepper, salt, and parmesan.
8. Divide risotto evenly on to two plates, add egg, and sprinkle with chives.
9. Serve and enjoy.
- **Nutrition Info:** Calories: 211; carbohydrates: 16.0g; protein: 12.0g; fat: 11.0g

276.Cheesy Green Chili Rice

Servings: 6 – 8 Servings
Cooking Time: 1 -2 Hours
Ingredients:
- 4-5 cups long-grain white rice, cooked
- 2 cans green chilies, diced
- 2 cups scallions, sliced thin
- 1 ½ cups plus 3 tablespoons Mozzarella cheese, grated
- 1 cup sour cream
- 2 tablespoons Parmesan cheese
- 1-2 tablespoons green hot sauce

Directions:

1. Place the rice and scallions in a large bowl and stir together.

2. In a separate bowl, combine sour cream, chilies with their juice, hot sauce and 1 ½ cups of the Mozzarella cheese.
3. Mix the cheese mixture into the rice.
4. Lightly spray the cooking pot with cooking spray. Add the rice mixture and press down to make sure it is in an even layer. Top with remaining Mozzarella and the Parmesan cheese.
5. Secure the lid and select slow cooking on high heat. Cook 1-2 hours or till bubbling hot and cheese is melted. Serve.

277.Salt-encrusted Prime Rib Roast

Servings: 8
Cooking Time: 45 Minutes
Ingredients:
- 2 cups salt
- 4 pounds prime rib roast
- 1 tablespoon black pepper

Directions:
1. Place in the ceramic pot the FoodiTM Cook &CrispTM reversible rack.
2. In a roasting pan that will fit in the Ninja Foodi, place the salt. Place the roast on top of the bed of salt. Season the pork with black pepper.
3. Place the pan with the meat on the rack.
4. Close the crisping lid and press the Bake/Roast button before pressing the START button.
5. Adjust the cooking time to 45 minutes.
- **Nutrition Info:** Calories: 382; Carbohydrates: 1.2g; Protein: 36.1g; Fat: 25.8g; Sugar: 0g; Sodium: 3092mg

278.Vegan-approved Fajita Pasta

Servings: 2
Cooking Time: 9 Minutes
Ingredients:
- 1 teaspoon oil
- 2 cloves of garlic, minced
- 1/3 cup chopped bell peppers
- 1/3 cup black beans, cooked
- 1/2 teaspoon taco seasoning mix
- 1 1/3 cups pasta, cooked according to package instruction
- 2/3 cup commercial enchilada sauce

- Salt and pepper to taste
Directions:
1. Press the sauté button on the Ninja Foodi and heat the oil. Stir in the garlic and bell peppers and allow to wilt for 3 minutes.
2. Add the rest of the ingredients.
3. Install pressure lid. Close Ninja Foodi, press the manual button, choose high settings, and set time to 6 minutes.
4. Once done cooking, do a quick release.
5. Serve and enjoy.
- **Nutrition Info:** Calories: 282; carbohydrates: 52.1g; protein: 10.4g; fat: 3.5g

279.Vegetable Masala Indian Style

Servings: 2
Cooking Time: 25 Minutes
Ingredients:
- 1 tablespoon olive oil
- 3 black whole peppercorns
- 2 green cardamoms
- 2 whole cloves
- 1 bay leave
- 1/4 cup tomato puree
- 1 teaspoon coriander powder
- 1/2 teaspoon garam masala
- ¼ teaspoon red chili powder
- 1/4 teaspoon turmeric powder
- 1/4 cup water
- 1/2 cup coconut milk
- ½ teaspoon sugar
- 1 small potato, peeled and chopped
- Salt and pepper to taste
- ¼ lemon, juiced
- 1 tablespoon chopped cilantro

Directions:
1. Press the sauté button on the Ninja Foodi and heat the oil.
2. Stir in the whole peppercorns, cardamoms, cloves, and bay leaf until fragrant.
3. Add in the tomato puree, coriander powder, garam masala, chili powder, and turmeric powder.
4. Stir in water, coconut milk, sugar and potatoes. Season with salt and pepper to taste.

5. Install pressure lid. Close Ninja Foodi, press the button, choose high settings, and set time to 20 minutes. Once done cooking, do a quick release.
6. Open the lid and stir in the lemon juice and cilantro. Serve and enjoy.

- **Nutrition Info:** Calories: 261; carbohydrates: 14g; protein: 4g; fat: 21g

280.Artichoke Dip

Servings: 6 Servings
Cooking Time: 6 Minutes
Ingredients:

- ¼ cup chicken broth
- 4 oz cream cheese
- 5 ounces chopped spinach
- 1 cup canned artichoke hearts
- ½ cup sour cream
- 1 clove garlic
- ½ tsp onion powder
- 6 ounces parmesan cheese, grated
- 6 ounces Swiss cheese

Directions:

1. Add all the ingredients to the Ninja Foodi Pot except the parmesan cheese and Swiss cheese.
2. Close the lid and set the steamer valve to seal. Use the pressure cooker function and cook the dip on high pressure for 4 minutes. Do a quick pressure release and open the pot.
3. Add the cheeses, reserving a small amount of each, and mix. Sprinkle the final cheese over the top of the dip and lower the crisper plate over the dip.
4. Use the broil function for 2 minutes to brown the cheese. Serve hot!

- **Nutrition Info:** Calories: 427g, Carbohydrates: 10g, Protein: 22g, Fat: 32g, Sugar: 2g, Sodium: 812mg

281.Cool Beet Chips

Servings: 8
Cooking Time: 8 Hours 10 Mins
Ingredients:

- ½ beet, peeled and sliced

Directions:

1. Arrange beet slices in single layer in the Cook and Crisp basket
2. Place the basket in the pot and close the crisping lid
3. Press the Dehydrate button and let it dehydrate for 8 hours at 135 degrees F
4. Once the dehydrating is done, remove the basket from pot and transfer slices to your Air Tight container, serve and enjoy!

- **Nutrition Info:** 35 calories, 0g fat, 8g carbs, 1g protein

282.Vegetarian-approved Meatballs In Bbq Sauce

Servings: 2
Cooking Time: 10 Minutes
Ingredients:

- ¼ cup water
- 1-pound frozen vegan meatballs
- 3/4 cup barbecue sauce
- 1/2 can cranberry sauce
- Salt and pepper to taste

Directions:

1. Place all ingredients in the Ninja Foodi and give a good stir.
2. Install pressure lid. Close Ninja Foodi, press the manual button, choose high settings, and set time to 10 minutes.
3. Once done cooking, do a quick release.
4. Serve and enjoy.

- **Nutrition Info:** Calories: 357; carbohydrates: 68.1g; protein: 17.1g; fat: 1.8g

283.Breakfast Oats With Apricots 'n Nuts

Servings: 2
Cooking Time: 6 Minutes
Ingredients:

- 1 ½ cups water
- 1 cup chopped strawberries, for topping
- 1 cup freshly squeezed orange juice
- 1 cup steel cut oats
- 1 tbsp chopped dried apricots
- 1 tbsp dried cranberries
- 1 tbsp raisins
- 1/4 tsp ground cinnamon
- 1/8 tsp salt
- 2 tbsp butter

- 2 tbsp pure maple syrup
- 3 tbsp chopped pecans, for topping

Directions:
1. Lightly grease Ninja Foodi insert with cooking spray and then add all ingredients except for pecans. Mix well.
2. Install pressure lid.
3. Close Ninja Foodi, press pressure button, choose high settings, and set time to 6 minutes.
4. Once done cooking, do a quick release.
5. Transfer to two bowl and evenly divide toppings on bowl.
6. Serve and enjoy.
- **Nutrition Info:** Calories: 507; carbohydrates: 72.4g; protein: 11.1g; fat: 19.2g

284.Ninja Foodi Cola Roast

Servings: 8
Cooking Time: 2 Hours
Ingredients:
- 4 pounds beef sirloin roast
- 1 can cola
- 3 cups water
- 1 clove of garlic, minced
- 1 bay leaf
- Salt and pepper to taste

Directions:
1. Place in the ceramic pot the FoodiTM Cook &CrispTM basket insert.
2. Place all ingredients in a bowl and allow the beef to soak in the cola for at least overnight.
3. Place the marinated beef in the basket insert.
4. Close the crisping lid and press the Bake/Roast button before pressing the START button.
5. Adjust the cooking time to 2 hours.
- **Nutrition Info:** Calories: 416; Carbohydrates: 12.7g; Protein: 38.8g; Fat: 23.3g; Sugar: 6.9g; Sodium: 736mg

285.Cheesy Artichoke & Crab Dip

Servings: 4 Cups
Cooking Time: 30 Minutes
Ingredients:
- 1 pound lump crab meat

- 14 ounce can artichoke hearts, drained
- ¾ cups cheddar cheese, grated
- 1/3 cup Parmesan cheese
- 6 tablespoons sour cream
- 6 tablespoons mayonnaise
- 2 tablespoons chives, chopped
- 1-2 teaspoons hot sauce
- 1 teaspoon lemon juice

Directions:
1. Chop the artichokes and crab and place them in a mixing bowl. Add the remaining ingredients and mix till combined. Transfer to a baking dish that will fit inside the cooking pot.
2. Add the Tender Crisp lid and lock into place. Set the temperature for 400 degrees and bake 30 minutes or till cheese is melted and top is golden brown.
3. Serve with your favorite chips, crackers or toasted bread

286.Crispy 'n Tasty Cauliflower Bites

Servings: 4
Cooking Time: 10 Minutes
Ingredients:
- 3 cloves of garlic, minced
- 1 tablespoon olive oil
- ½ teaspoon salt
- ½ teaspoon smoked paprika
- 4 cups cauliflower florets

Directions:
1. Place in the ceramic pot the FoodiTM Cook &CrispTM basket.
2. Place all ingredients in a bowl and toss to combine.
3. Place the seasoned cauliflower florets in the basket.
4. Close the crisping lid and press the Air Crisp button before pressing the START button.
5. Adjust the cooking time to 10 minutes.
6. Give the basket a shake for even cooking
- **Nutrition Info:** Calories: 130; Carbohydrates: 12.4g; Protein: 4.3g; Fat: 7g; Sugar: 0.7g; Sodium: 642mg

287.Spicy Short Ribs

Servings: 4
Cooking Time: 60 Minutes

Ingredients:

- 2 teaspoons canola oil
- 1 onion, diced
- 4 cloves of garlic, minced
- 2 pounds beef short ribs
- 1 teaspoon paprika
- 1 teaspoon cumin
- 2 tablespoons apple cider vinegar
- 1 can cola
- 1 tablespoon raspberry jam
- 1 tablespoon Worcestershire sauce
- 1 tablespoon sugar
- 2 tablespoons cornstarch
- 2 tablespoons water
- Salt and pepper to taste

Directions:

1. Press the Sear/Sauté button and then the START button. Heat the oil and sauté the onion and garlic until fragrant.
2. Stir in the beef short ribs and season with salt, pepper, paprika, and cumin.
3. Stir until all sides are lightly golden.
4. Add in the apple cider vinegar, cola, raspberry jam, Worcestershire sauce, and sugar.
5. Close the pressure lid and set the vent to SEAL.
6. Press the Pressure button and adjust the cooking time to 60 minutes.
7. Do quick pressure release. Once the lid is open, press the Sear/Sauté button and stir in the cornstarch slurry. Allow to simmer until the sauce thickens.
- **Nutrition Info:** Calories: 471; Carbohydrates: 45.1g; Protein: 22g; Fat: 22.5g; Sugar: 21.9g; Sodium: 624mg

288.Scalloped Pineapple

Servings: 8 – 10 Servings
Cooking Time: 35 Minutes
Ingredients:

- 20 ounce can pineapple tidbits, reserve ¼ cup juice,
- 20 ounce can crushed pineapple, drained
- 40 Ritz crackers, crushed
- 2 cups sharp cheddar cheese, grated
- ½ cup sugar
- ½ cup butter, melted

- 6 tablespoons flour

Directions:

1. In a mixing bowl, combine all ingredients except the cracker crumbs and the butter.
2. Lightly spray the cooking pot with cooking spray. Add the pineapple mixture.
3. In a small bowl, combine the crackers crumbs and butter. Sprinkle over the top of the pineapple mixture.
4. Add the Tender Crisp lid and set the temperature to 350 degrees. Bake 35 minutes or till top is golden brown. Serve warm.

289.Garden Fresh Veggie Combo

Servings: 5
Cooking Time: 35 Minutes
Ingredients:

- 6 tsp. olive oil, divided
- ½ lb. carrots, peeled and sliced
- 2 lb. zucchini, sliced
- 1 tbsp. fresh basil, chopped
- Salt and freshly ground black pepper, to taste

Directions:

1. In a bowl, mix together 2 tsp. of oil and carrots.
2. Arrange the "Cook & Crisp Basket" in the pot of Ninja Foodi.
3. Close the Ninja Foodi with crisping lid and select "Air Crisp".
4. Press "Start/Stop" to begin and set the temperature to 400 degrees F.
5. Set the time for 5 minutes to preheat.
6. Now, place the carrots into "Cook & Crisp Basket".
7. Close the Ninja Foodi with crisping lid and select "Air Crisp".
8. Set the temperature to 400 degrees F for 5 minutes. Press "Start/Stop" to begin.
9. Meanwhile, in a large bowl, mix together remaining oil, zucchini, basil, salt and black pepper.
10. Open the lid and place the zucchini mixture into basket with carrots.
11. Close the Ninja Foodi with crisping lid and set the time for 30 minutes.

12. Press "Start/Stop" to begin. Toss the vegetable mixture 2-3 times during the coking. Open the lid and serve.
- **Nutrition Info:** Calories: 96; Carbohydrates: 10.6g; Protein: 2.6g; Fat: 5.9g; Sugar: 5.4g; Sodium: 80mg; Fiber: 3.1g

290.Vanilla-espresso Flavored Oats

Servings: 2
Cooking Time: 20 Minutes
Ingredients:
- 1/2 cup milk
- 1/2 cup steel cut oats
- 1 teaspoon espresso powder
- 1/4 teaspoon salt
- 1 1/4 cups water
- 1 tablespoon sugar
- 1 teaspoon vanilla extract
- Finely grated chocolate

Directions:
1. Mix well salt, espresso powder, sugar, oats, milk, and water in Ninja Foodi.
2. Install pressure lid and place valve to vent position.
3. Close Ninja Foodi, press steam button, and set time to 2 minutes.
4. Once done cooking, do a natural release for 10-minutes and then do a quick release.
5. Uncover pot and stir in vanilla extract. Spoon into bowls.
6. Garnish with grated chocolate.
7. Serve and enjoy.
- **Nutrition Info:** Calories: 198; carbohydrates: 27.6g; protein: 6.5g; fat: 6.8g

291.Lamb Marsala

Servings: 2 Servings
Cooking Time: 1 Hour 40 Minutes
Ingredients:
- 2 lamb shanks
- 1 cup chicken stock
- 2/3 cup Marsala wine
- 1 onion, chopped
- 8 cloves garlic, halved
- 4 bay leaves
- 2 tablespoons tomato paste
- 2 twigs rosemary
- Salt & pepper to taste

- Olive oil

Directions:
1. Trim off the excess fat from the lamb. Rub them with salt and pepper.
2. Set the cooker to sauté on med-high heat and add a splash of olive oil. When the oil is hot add the onions and garlic and cook till almost translucent, stirring often. Stir in the tomato paste and cook 2-3 minutes more.
3. Add lamb shanks, one at a time, and brown on both sides. Add both shanks to the pot, making sure they are meat side down. Add the bay leaves, wine, rosemary and chicken stock and bring to a boil.
4. Secure the lid and select pressure cooking on high. Set the timer for 45 minutes.
5. When the timer goes off, use quick release to remove the lid. Flip the lamb and secure the lid again. Cook another 25 minutes.
6. Quick release the lid and set the cooker back to sauté on medium heat. Cook another 10 – 15 minutes till the sauce is thick and sticky, being sure to glaze the lamb every few minutes. Serve.

292.Steamed Lemon Grass Crab Legs

Servings: 4
Cooking Time: 25 Minutes
Ingredients:
- 2 tablespoons vegetable oil
- 3 cloves of garlic, minced
- 1 piece fresh ginger root, crushed
- 1 stalk lemon grass, crushed
- 2 tablespoons fish sauce
- 1 tablespoon oyster sauce
- 2 pounds frozen Alaskan king crab
- Salt and pepper to taste

Directions:
1. Place the FoodiTM Cook &CrispTM reversible rack inside the ceramic pot.
2. Pour water into the pot.
3. Combine all ingredients in a big Ziploc bag and marinate for at least 30 minutes.
4. Place the crabs on the reversible rack.
5. Close the pressure lid and set the vent to SEAL.
6. Press the Steam button and adjust the cooking time to 25 minutes.

- **Nutrition Info:** Calories: 564; Carbohydrates: 5.3g; Protein: 89.1g; Fat: 20.7g; Sugar: 2.2g; Sodium: 1023mg

293.Asian Spiced Chicken Wings

Servings: 2 Servings
Cooking Time: 30 Mins
Ingredients:
- 8 chicken wings
- 2 tablespoons soy sauce
- 2 tablespoons Chinese spice
- Salt & pepper

Directions:
1. Add the soy sauce, spice, salt and pepper to a large mixing bowl and stir to combine.
2. Add the wings and toss to coat well.
3. Place the rack in the bottom of the cooker. Place the chicken on it and pour any remaining sauce over it.
4. Add the Tender Crisp lid and set the temperature to 350 degrees.
5. Cook for 15 minutes, then turn the chicken over and cook another 15 minutes. Serve with your favorite dipping sauce.

294.Bacon Cheeseburger Dip

Servings: 8 Servings
Cooking Time: 30 Mins
Ingredients:
- 1 pound ground beef
- 1 package cream cheese, soft
- 2 cups cheddar cheese , grated
- 10 ounce can of Rotel tomatoes with green chilies
- 1 cup sour cream
- 2/3 cup bacon, cooked crisp and crumbled

Directions:
1. Set the cooker to the sauté function on med-high. Add ground beef and cook through, breaking it up while cooking. Drain the fat.
2. Combine remaining ingredients in a large bowl and mix till well combined. Stir in ground beef.
3. Pour into a baking dish that will fit inside the cooking pot. Add the Tender Crisp lid and lock into place.
4. Set the temperature to 350 degrees. Bake for 20 – 25 minutes or hot and bubbly.

5. Serve with your favorite chips or crackers for dipping.

295.Roasted Whole Chicken

Servings:4
Cooking Time: 60 Minutes
Ingredients:
- ½ cup salt
- 10 cups water
- 2 pounds whole rotisserie chicken
- 1 sprig rosemary
- 1 tablespoon sage

Directions:
1. Dissolve the salt in water to make a brine in a deep bowl or stock pot.
2. Soak the chicken and put in the rosemary and sage.
3. Allow the chicken to marinate in the brine for overnight.
4. Place in the ceramic pot the FoodiTM Cook & CrispTM reversible rack.
5. Place the chicken on the rack.
6. Close the crisping lid and press the Bake/Roast button before pressing the START button.
7. Adjust the cooking time to 1hour.
- **Nutrition Info:** Calories: 406; Carbohydrates: 0.9g; Protein: 34.2g; Fat: 29.5g; Sugar: 0g; Sodium: 899mg

296.Cheesy Cauliflower

Servings: 5
Cooking Time: 35 Minutes
Ingredients:
- 1 tbsp. prepared mustard
- 1 head cauliflower
- 1 tsp. avocado mayonnaise
- ½ c. grated Parmesan cheese
- ¼ c. butter, chopped

Directions:
1. Press "Sauté" on Ninja Foodi and add butter and cauliflower.
2. Sauté for about 3 minutes and add rest of the ingredients.
3. Lock the lid and set the Ninja Foodi to "Pressure" for about 30 minutes.
4. Release the pressure naturally and dish out to serve hot.

- **Nutrition Info:** 155 calories, 13.3g fat, 3.8g carbs, 6.7g protein

297.Crab Frittata

Servings: 4 Servings
Cooking Time: 50 Mins
Ingredients:
- 2 cups lump crabmeat
- 4 eggs
- 1 cup half and half
- 1 cup Parmesan cheese, grated
- 1 cup green onions, chopped
- 1 teaspoon salt
- 1 teaspoon pepper
- 1 teaspoon sweet smoked paprika
- 1 teaspoon Italian seasoning

Directions:
1. Whisk egg and half-and-half together in a large bowl. Add seasonings and Parmesan and stir to mix.
2. Stir in the onions and crab meat.
3. Wrap some foil around the base of a springform pan that will fit inside the cooking pot. Pour the egg mixture into the pan.
4. Place the rack in the pot and add 2 cups of water. Place the pan on the rack and secure the lid. Select pressure cooking on high and set the timer for 40 minutes.
5. When the timer goes off, let sit for 10 minutes. Then use quick release to remove the lid. Carefully remove the pan and remove the outer ring. Serve warm or at room temperature.

298.Steamed Mussels With Fennel And Tomatoes

Servings: 8
Cooking Time: 15 Minutes
Ingredients:
- 2 shallots, chopped
- 4 cloves of garlic, chopped
- 1 bulb fennel, sliced
- 1 tomato, cubed
- ½ cup white wine
- ½ cup heavy cream
- 4 pounds mussels, cleaned
- 1/3 cup basil leaves, torn

- Salt to taste

Directions:
1. Place everything in a large Ziploc bag and allow the mussels to soak in the marinade.
2. Place the FoodiTM Cook &CrispTM reversible rack inside the ceramic pot.
3. Pour water into the pot.
4. Place the mussels and the vegetables (except the marinade) on the reversible rack.
5. Close the pressure lid and set the vent to SEAL.
6. Press the Steam button and adjust the cooking time to 15 minutes.
7. Meanwhile, pour the marinade on a saucepan and heat over medium flame until the sauce thickens.
8. Serve the sauce over the clams.
- **Nutrition Info:** Calories: 270; Carbohydrates: 15.7g; Protein: 16.3g; Fat: 15.7g; Sugar: ,4.7g; Sodium: 245mg

299.Summertime Mousse

Servings: 2
Cooking Time: 12 Minutes
Ingredients:
- 4-oz. cream cheese, softened
- ½ C. heavy cream
- 2 tbsp. fresh lemon juice
- 2 tbsp. honey
- 2 pinches salt

Directions:
1. Select "Bake/Roast" of Ninja Foodi and set the temperature to 350 degrees F.
2. Press "Start/Stop" to begin and preheat the Ninja Foodi for about 10 minutes.
3. In a bowl, add all the ingredients and mix until well combined.
4. Transfer the mixture into 2 ramekins.
5. In the pot of Ninja Foodi, arrange the ramekins.
6. Close the Ninja Foodi with crisping lid and set the time for 12 minutes.
7. Press "Start/Stop" to begin.
8. Open the lid and set the ramekins aside to cool.
9. Refrigerate for at least 3 hours before serving.

- **Nutrition Info:** Calories per serving: 369; Carbohydrates: 20g; Protein: 5.1g; Fat: 31g; Sugar: 17.7g; Sodium: 338mg; Fiber: 0.1g

300.Luncheon Green Beans

Servings: 4
Cooking Time: 15 Minutes
Ingredients:
- 1 lb. fresh green beans
- 2 tbsps. butter
- 1 minced garlic clove
- Salt and freshly ground black pepper
- 1½ c. water

Directions:
1. Put all the ingredients in the pot of Ninja Foodi and lock the lid.
2. Press "Pressure" and cook for about 5 minutes.
3. Release the pressure quickly and dish out to serve hot.
- **Nutrition Info:** 87 calories, 5.9g fat, 8.4g carbs, 2.2g protein

CPSIA information can be obtained
at www.ICGtesting.com
Printed in the USA
LVHW020734090121
675855LV00009B/445